From c[...] learn to cut and style hair with the detailed instructions and helpful line drawings in this book. You'll look great—and save on trips to the hairdresser—with advice on . . .

BANGS · SECTIONING · LAYERING · FEATHERING · PRE-PERM CUTTING · STRAIGHTENING WAVES · BEVELING · THINNING · TAPERING
and more!

HAIRCUTTING AT HOME

HAIRCUTTING AT HOME

John R. Albano

BERKLEY BOOKS, NEW YORK

HAIRCUTTING AT HOME

A Berkley Book / published by arrangement with
the author

PRINTING HISTORY
Berkley edition / April 1995

ISBN: 0-425-14688-X

BERKLEY®
Berkley Books are published by The Berkley Publishing Group,
200 Madison Avenue, New York, New York 10016.
BERKLEY and the "B" design
are trademarks belonging to Berkley Publishing Corporation.

PRINTED IN THE UNITED STATES OF AMERICA

10 9 8 7 6 5 4 3 2 1

Contents

HAIRCUTTING AT HOME

Introduction

Anyone can give a basic haircut to a man, woman, or child by following the few elementary techniques explained in this book. With some practice, you can give a basic haircut like a professional and save a bundle of money while doing it. If you can hold a scissors and comb in your hands, you are halfway there—just follow the easy steps and illustrations as we go along.

I have been cutting hair for twenty-seven years (seventeen in my own full-service salon for men, women, and children). I have probably given over one hundred thousand haircuts in that time and have figured out the shortcuts (no pun intended) and easiest and best ways to cut hair.

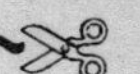 1

The Perfect Face

The Oval Face

The most flattering shape of face is an oval. With this shape, any haircut will look good, whether styled back, in a side part, or with bangs. However, some of us are not blessed with this type of face. As the stylist, you have to make a decision on which way your client looks best. We are able to remold the face by way of the hair.

Place your client in front of a mirror. What is the shape of the face? Is it round, square, long, or thin? Where would he or she benefit with more/less weight? With more volume on top? Fuller on the sides? Combed back? Combed down? Off-center part? Center part? Comb the hair in different ways and observe what looks best. Then, design this look into your cut. By thinking of hair as weight as opposed to length, and designing the style along these lines, we can create the illusion of an oval.

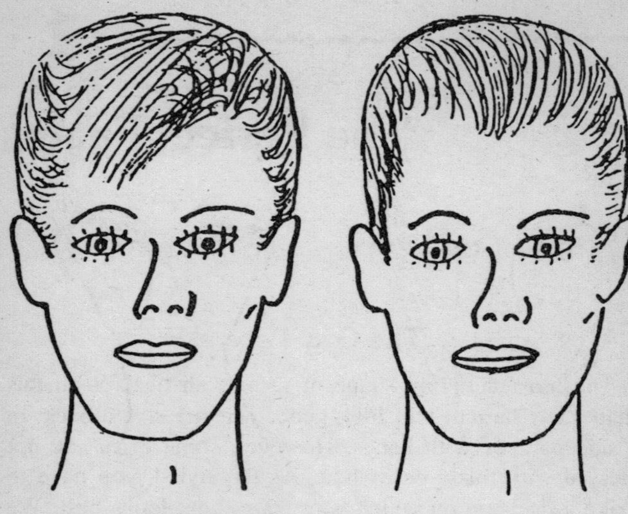

Long face made more attractive by hairstyle

Long face in less attractive hairstyle

The Long Face

A long face will look more attractive if the hair is combed down over the forehead in bangs or with a side part and combed across the head, with some weight at the sides.

A long face will not benefit with the hair off the forehead, too full on top, or styled back.

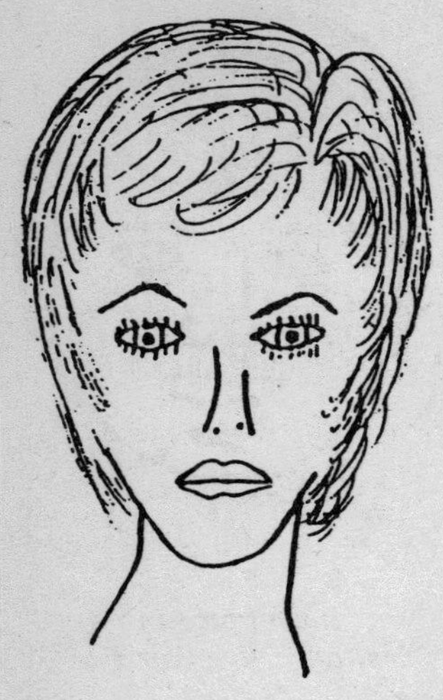

Triangular face made more attractive by hairstyle

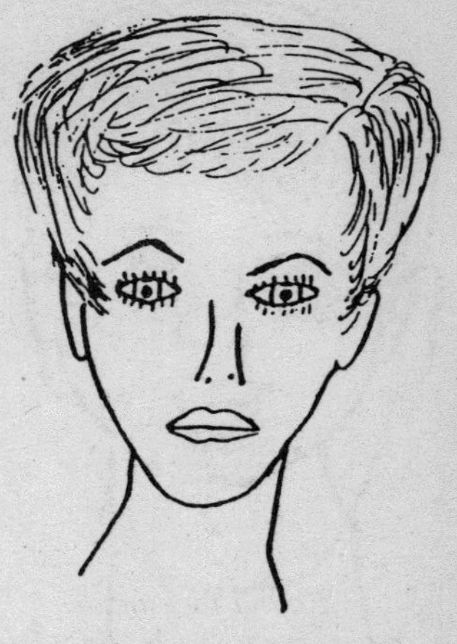

Triangular face in less attractive hairstyle

The Triangular Face

A side part across the forehead with weight on the lower sides will work here.

Fullness on the top and upper sides or hair off the face will only exaggerate the narrow chin.

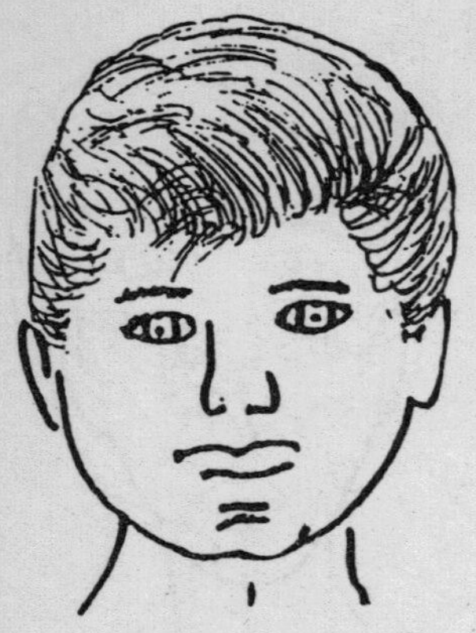

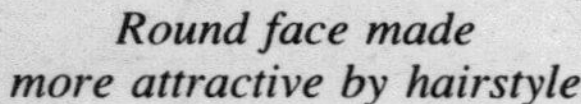

Round face made more attractive by hairstyle

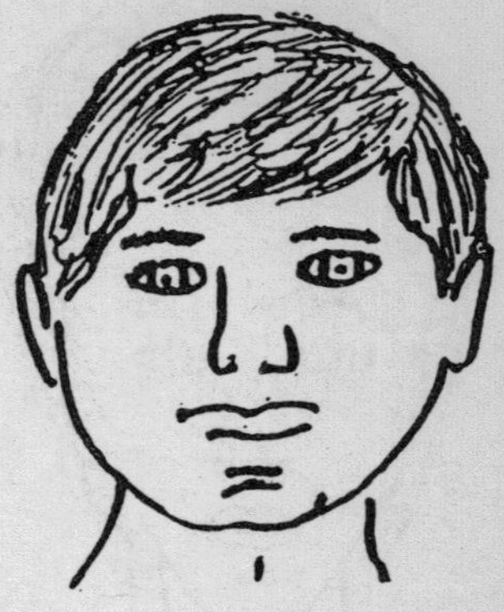

Round face in less attractive hairstyle

The Round Face

A round face looks best with volume on top, off the face, and tighter on the sides.

Hair styled forward and/or flat on top will only add to the roundness of the face.

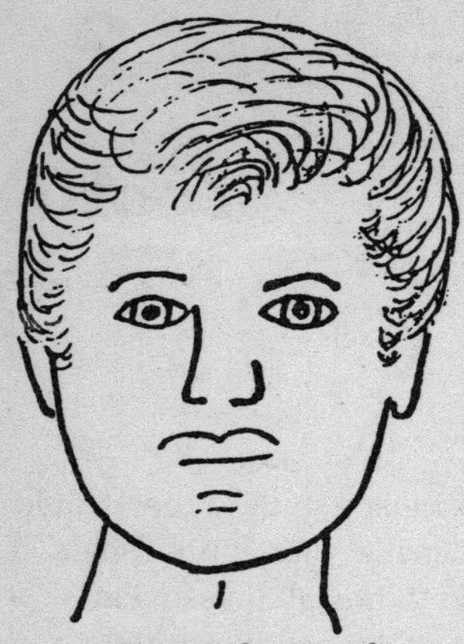

Square face made more attractive by hairstyle

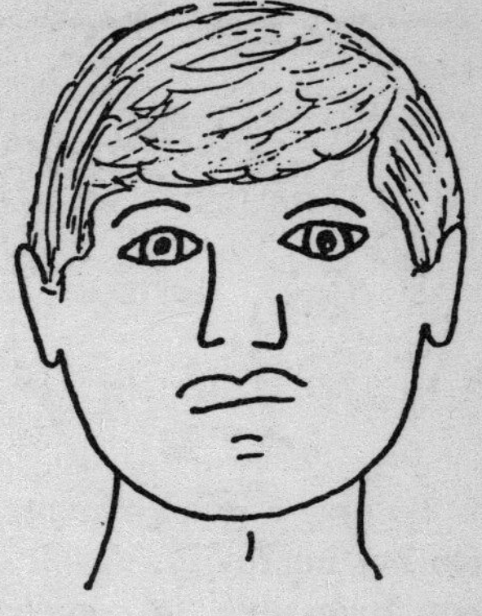

Square face in less attractive hairstyle

The Square Face

Volume on top, off the face, and some weight at the sides will be good here. An equal distribution of weight is a plus.

Too flat on top and too close on the sides will only accentuate the square look.

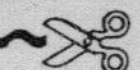

2

Tools

To give a good haircut, you must use the proper tools. Do not improvise; it will only make your job difficult, if not impossible, to complete. A nominal investment is a must, but you will save plenty of money every time you cut a family member's hair.

Haircutting Shears

There are many styles and sizes, but I prefer one about five to six inches long (that is a moderate length). You do not have to spend a lot of money on a pair of shears, but don't buy the cheapest pair you can find. Move only the thumb when cutting. Practice this movement before beginning.

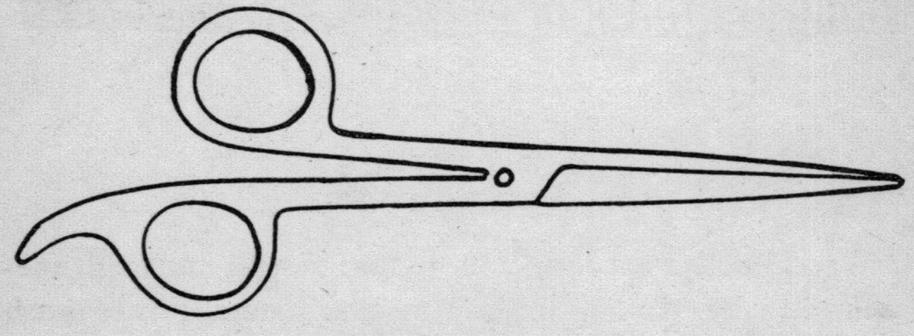

Haircutting shears

Thinning Shears

Used on 80 percent of cuts, these tools are a must for a good haircut. A lot of hairstylists do not even use this useful tool. You can correct mistakes and make many a haircut look light and airy, not heavy and matted.

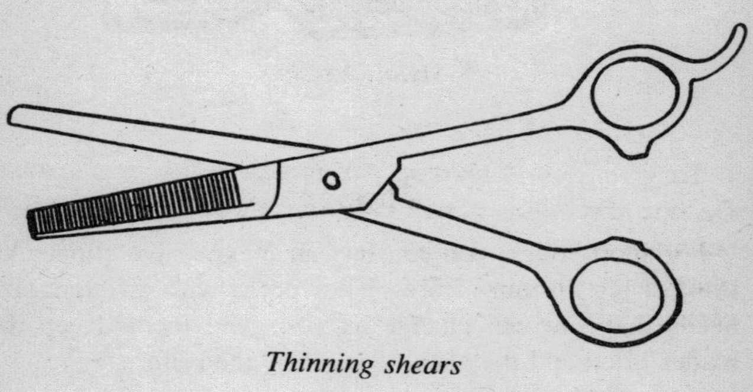

Thinning shears

Comb

A good rubber comb about seven to eight inches in length is best. Many different styles and sizes are available.

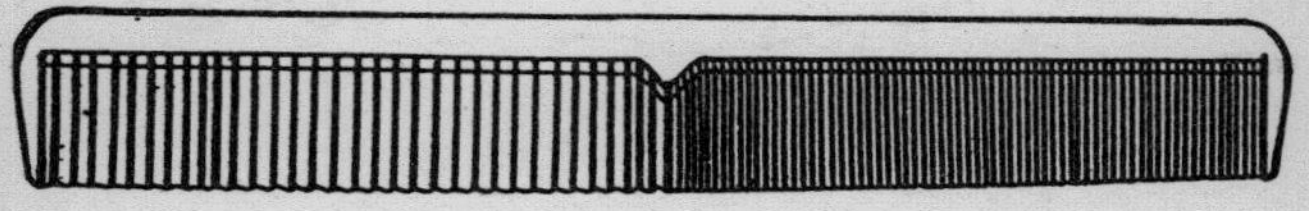

Comb

Styling Brush

Try to select a brush with nylon bristles and with medium density. A conventional brush or natural bristle brush has bristles too close together and stays only on the top layer of hair. A nylon bristle brush, on the other hand, will get into all layers of hair, a must for today's hairstyles.

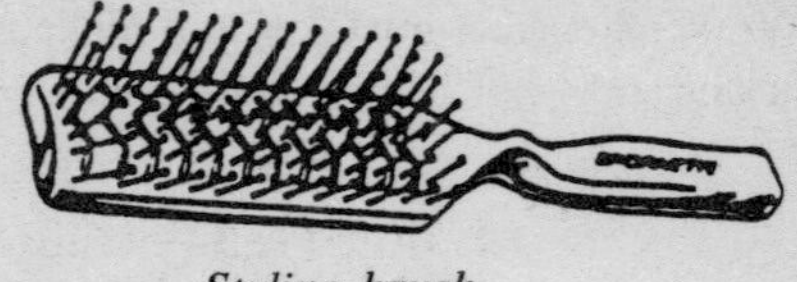

Styling brush

Clipper

For short styles, you can buy an inexpensive clipper kit in most big discount stores. They come with different size heads that you can change as you need them. Keep the blades oiled and they will do a very good job.

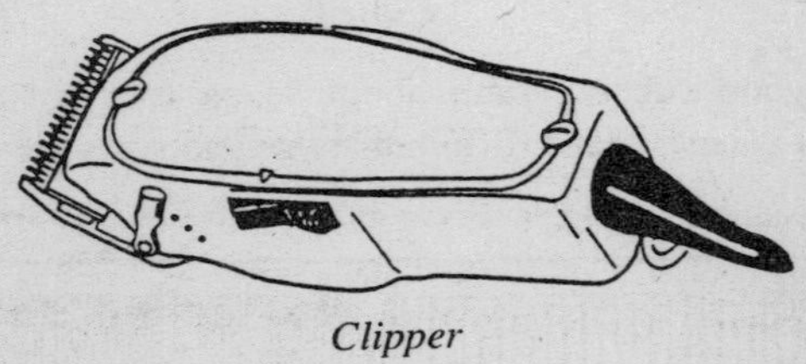

Clipper

Trimmer

This very important tool is used on most, if not all, layered haircuts. A trimmer is like a clipper, but it will cut very close—almost razor close—for a finished look for short styles. Some clipper kits include a trimmer or trimmer attachment.

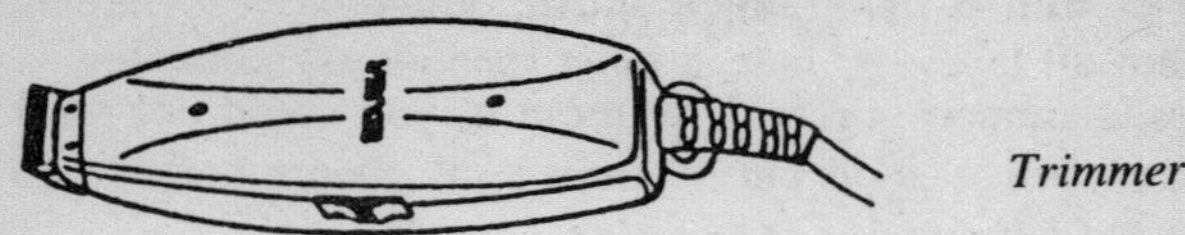

Trimmer

Duster Brush and Haircutting Cape

These can be found in a beauty supply store. A duster brush is a soft brush to clean the hair away as you work, so you can see what you are doing as you go along. A haircutting cape with a velcro collar keeps hair off the client.

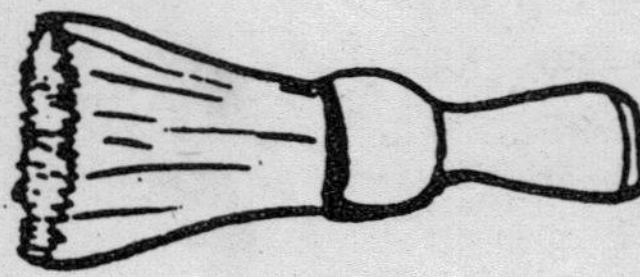

Duster brush

Blow-Dryer

Obviously, a blow-dryer is used to dry wet hair, but this useful tool has additional uses such as adding fullness or eliminating a stubborn curl, as we will see later.

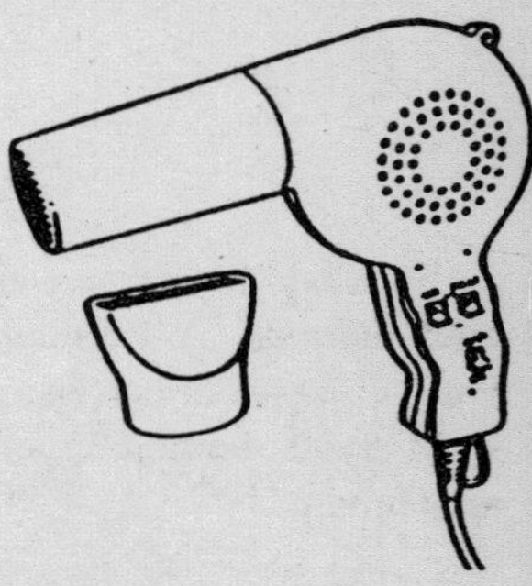

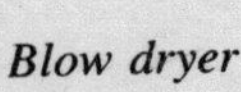

Blow dryer

Shampoo

Yes, shampoo is a tool. Without it, you could not relax the hair. For a good cut, shampoo all clients before you begin the haircut.

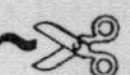 3

Techniques

Start With an Idea

Picture the finished haircut in your head before you begin. Many a haircutter started with good intentions but ended up with a mess because he didn't have a picture of the finished product in his head. Have some idea of what you want to do before you make the first cut. Talk to your client and see what she would like for herself, and ask about overall length, length on the sides, top, front, and back.

Your Fingers Are Your Guide

Fingers dictate the entire cut; the shears are only the finality of finger movement. Essentially, all short to medium-length layered haircuts use the same procedure, the difference being how long or short the hair is left at certain sections.

Take your time and go slowly. You will be amazed at the speed you will pick up in a short time.

Hair Maps

Hair maps were created as an aid to help you see how a certain cut would look if the hair were held straight out from the head (see the illustration on page 15). As you cut your sections, have in your mind the hair map for the cut you are doing. Hair maps will be used throughout this book to guide you along.

Caution: Know where the point of your shears is at all times.

Design Line

Design line is a term you will see many times in this book. Every haircut has one: long hair, short hair, and every length in between. It is the essence of every haircut. It is a line along the extreme bottom perimeter of the haircut.

The Ninety-Degree Rule: (Section-Section-Strip Method)

When cutting hair, the easiest way to give a haircut is by sections. Step by step, section by section, taking one section at a time until the haircut is finished. In this manner, you have the most control over what you are doing.

When cutting sections, we break the sections down into section strips, cutting section strips as you lift with your fingers or cut scissors over comb, as later described. You must *lift the hair out and away from the head at a ninety-degree angle* to the head, each and every time you cut. You regulate the length of the sections by how close or far from the scalp you hold your fingers (or comb) while cutting.

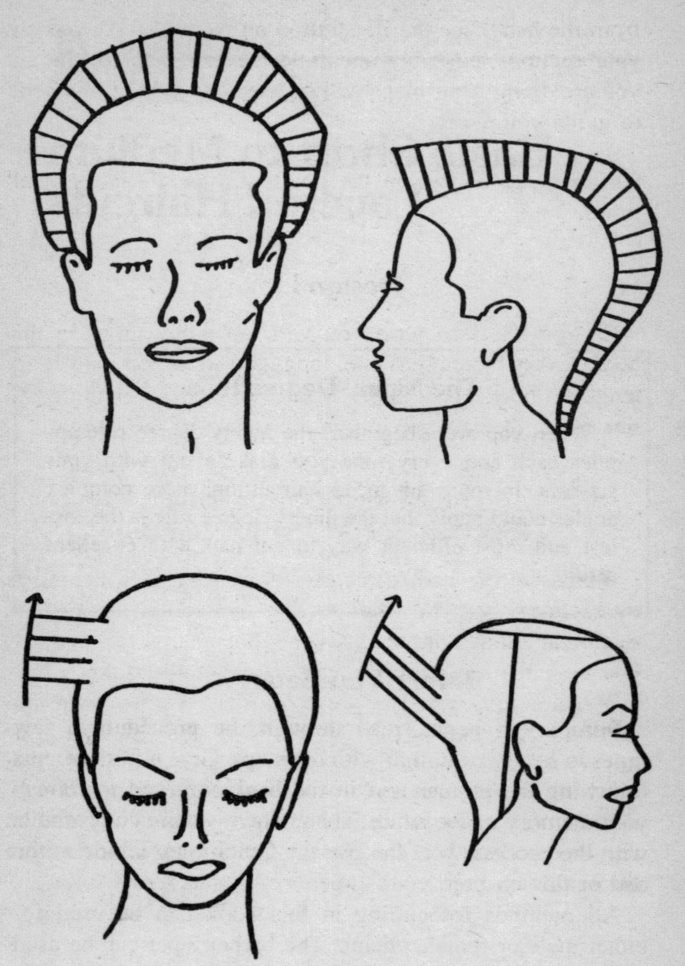

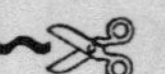 4

Basic Short to Medium Layered Haircuts

The Ninety-Degree Rule

When you are a beginner, the ninety-degree rule applies each and every time you make a cut with your scissors. In more advanced haircutting, more complex angles could apply, but the ninety-degree rule is the easiest and most efficient way to cut hair with excellent results.

Before You Begin . . .

Before you begin, read through the procedure a few times to become familiar with the steps. Give a few haircuts following the regular text in the beginning and to refresh your memory in the future. Then, when you are comfortable with the process, you can use the Quick Step Guide at the end of this chapter.

All methods for cutting in this book can be used for either male or female clients. The barber taper can be used on female cuts and the one-length all-around cut on male heads. It is up to you as the haircutter to determine the method and cut used and for whom.

Our First Cut

A basic short to medium layered haircut is a good place to start. It will teach you the basic movement of most haircuts, male or female.

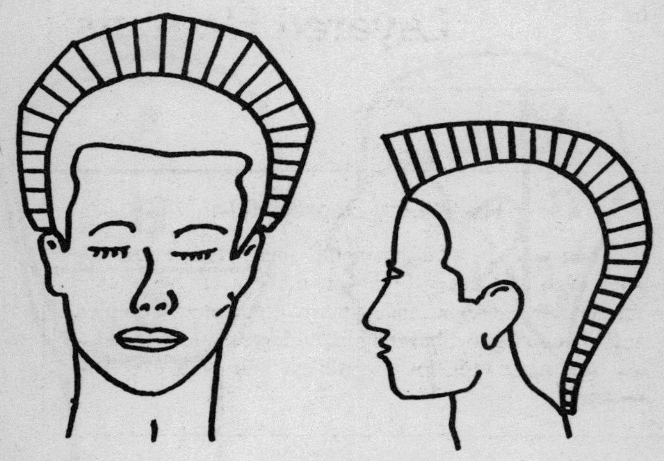

Our first cut

All sections are shown before cutting has begun.

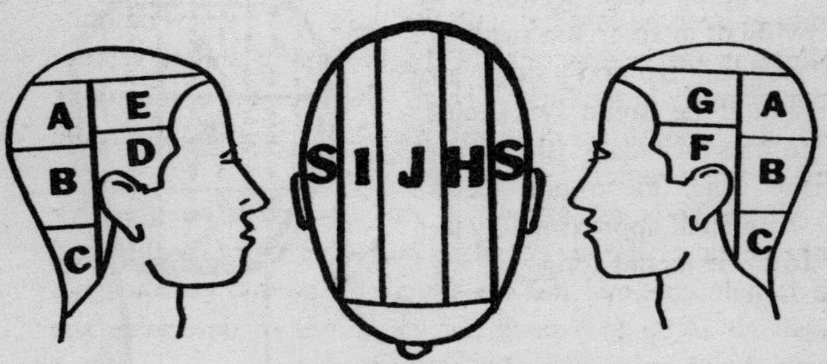

S designates side caps

Shampoo the hair and towel it to take most of the wetness out, but leave it moist. We will take one section at a time.

First, section the back of the head as shown. If the hair is too short to section, imagine where the sections should be.

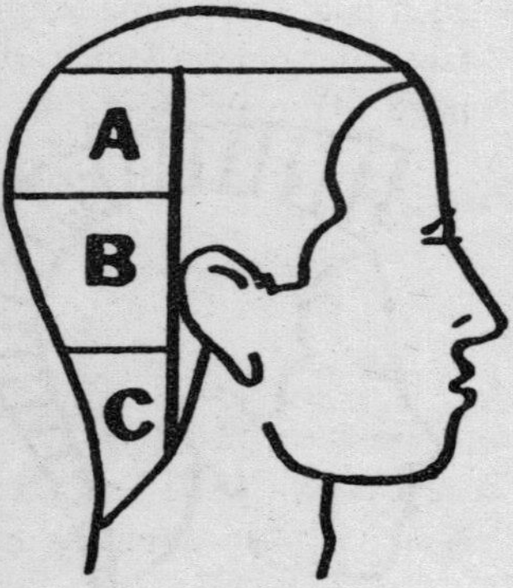

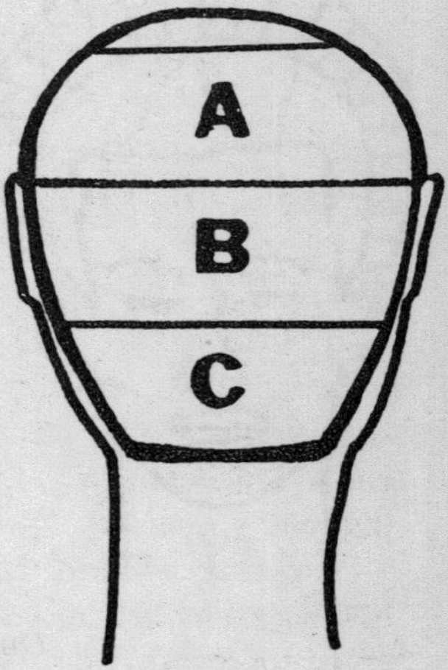

Section the back of the head

Out of these sections, we will cut in six to ten strips per section. Section strip size should be about one-quarter to one inch wide (the shorter the hair, the more section strips) and approximately two to three inches long.

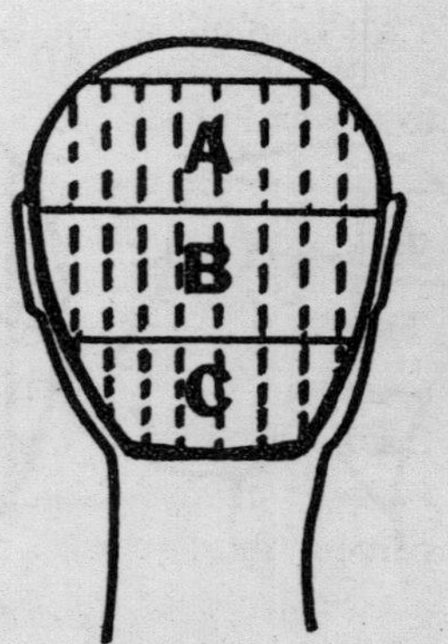

Section strips

Section A

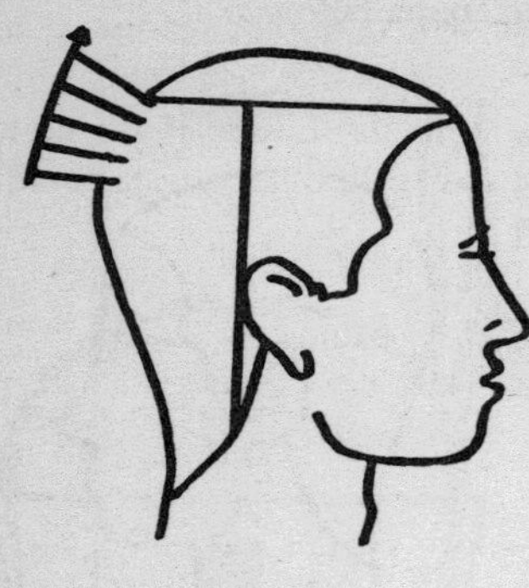

Section A

Start with the back right of section A. *Lift* the hair with the comb and, with your fingers at a ninety-degree angle out and away from the head each and every time you cut (see the ninety-degree rule, page 14), make your cut.

Length will vary depending on the overall length and style you want. Be careful in the crown area. Too short a cut will make the hair stand up on most heads (unless that's the look you want).

Now proceed to the next strip to the left of the first one, holding some hair in your fingers from the first strip as a guide for length. Make your cut, but don't forget to lift the hair at a ninety-degree angle out and away from the head.

Continue across all of section A, picking up strip by strip to the end of section A.

Section B

Pick up the first section strip in section B and a bit of section A for a length guide. Proceed in the same manner from right to left across section B, pulling hair out and away as always. Make the cut in section B about 20 to 30 percent shorter than section A, angling with your fingers, longer at the top of the cut and shorter at the bottom, for more of a tapered look. You can also leave this area longer, depending on your cut. (See hair maps below.)

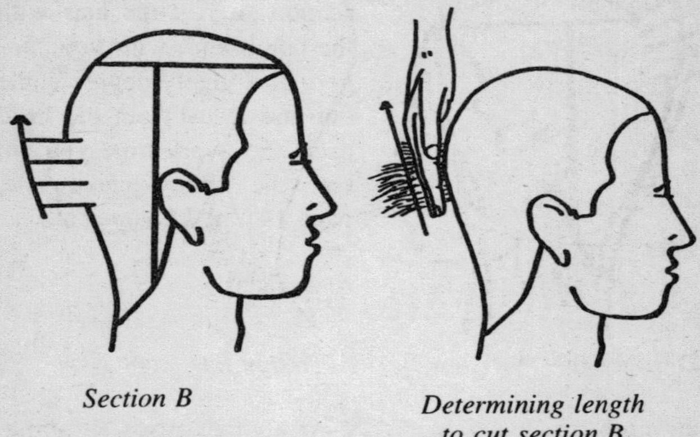

Section B

Determining length to cut section B

Section C

Next, pick up the first section C strip and proceed in the same manner as in the previous sections, again angling with your fingers so that the hair is shorter at the neck for the tapered look, or leave length as desired. You may tilt the head forward for a more comfortable cutting angle, but be careful to observe the ninety-degree rule.

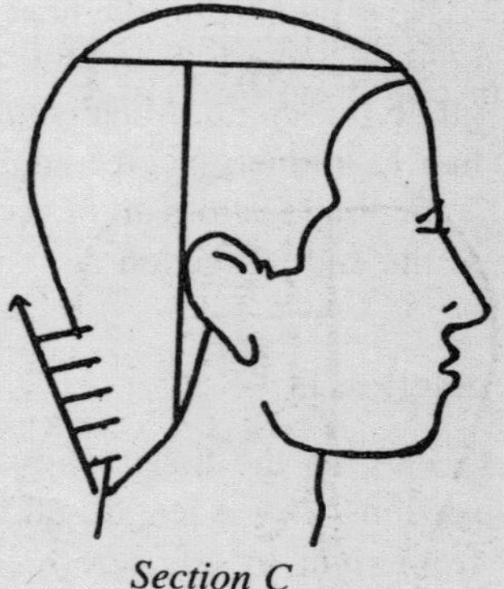

Section C

Design Line: Comb hair down and cut a design line at the nape area and sides of the neck with scissors, or you can

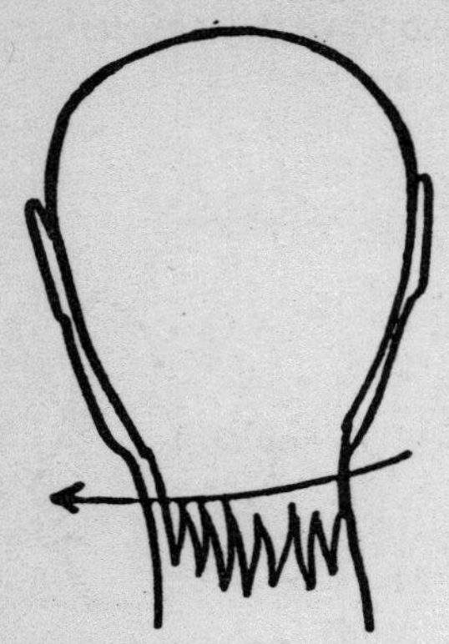

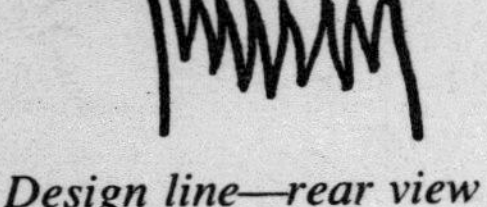

Design line—rear view

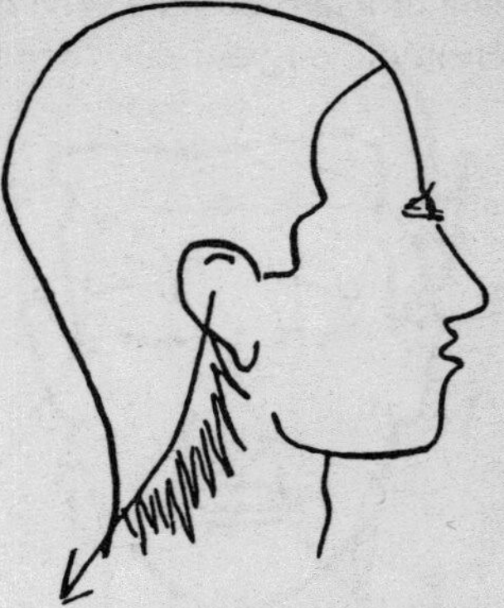

Design line—side view

use your trimmer if hair is short enough. (See finishing section on page 32.)

Section D

Section the right side, and either comb away section E or clip it out of the way.

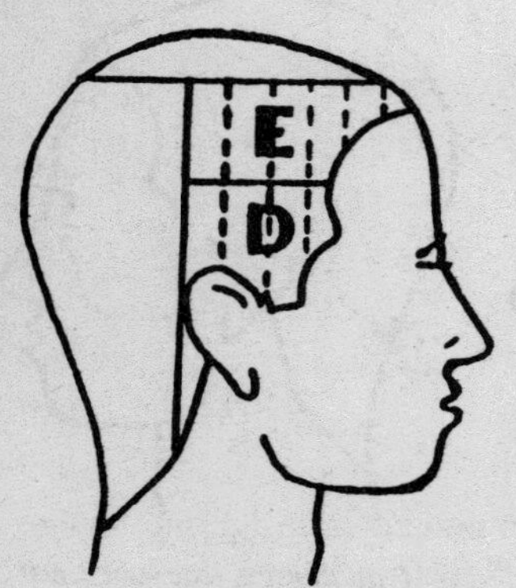

Section the right side

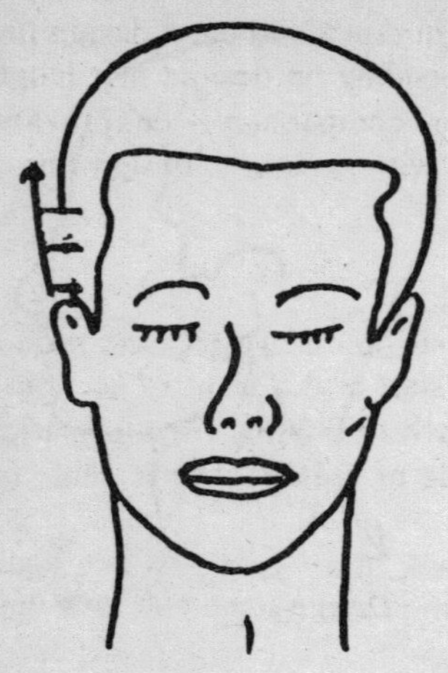

Section D

Starting from the front, hold the first section strip with fingers out and away at a ninety-degree angle and shorter toward the bottom. Make your first cut of section D and continue back, strip by strip, to sections B and C. Blend section D with sections B and C.

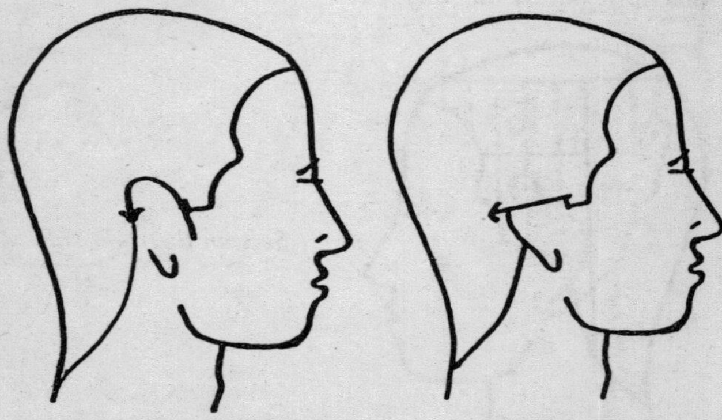

Cut design line around ear *Cut design line over ear*

Comb section D hair straight down and cut a design line around the ear or over it, depending on desired hair length (two lengths are shown for comparison—see previous page). Blend this design line with neck area design line.

Section E

Pin or comb side cap and section I away. Comb section E down over section D and start at the front of section E with the usual one-quarter-inch to one-inch section strips, holding in your fingers a little of section D as a guide for length.

Depending on length desired, make your first cut, again holding hair out away from the head as you cut, with hair a bit longer on top of cut. Continue back with one-quarter-inch to one-inch section strips to and into sections A and B. Comb hair forward at front of sections D and E and trim off excess.

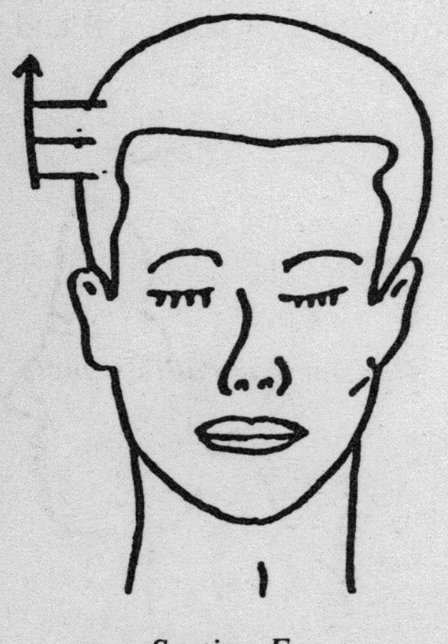

Section E

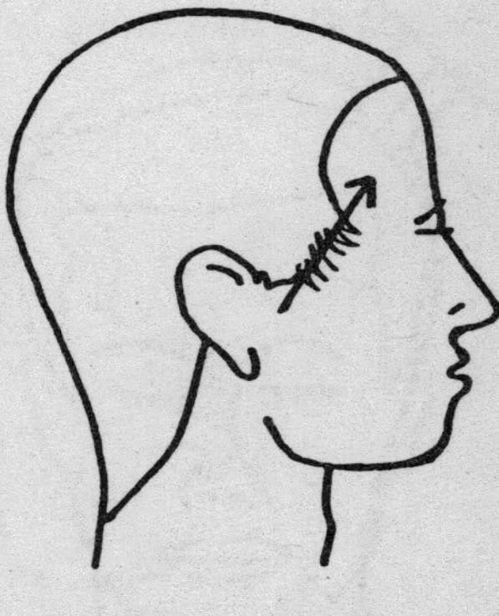

Comb hair of section E forward and trim excess

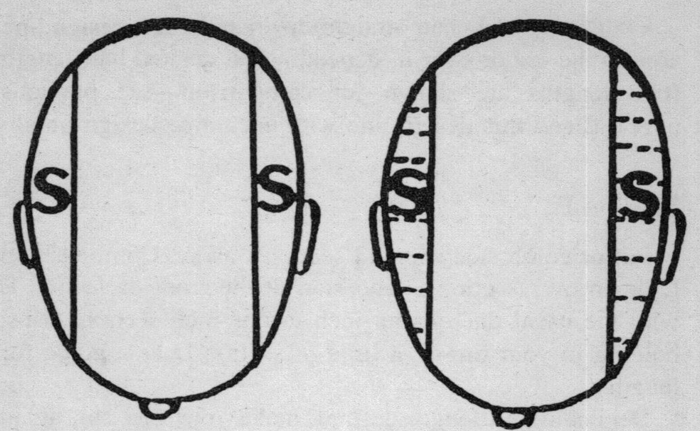

Side caps *Side caps sectioned*

Side Cap

The side cap sections (designated by S) are on both sides of the head, directly above section E and section G. These

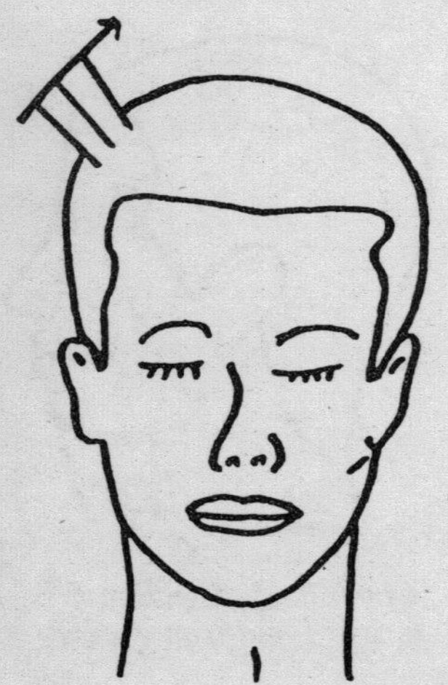

Cut side caps at this angle

side cap sections vary in width on every haircut you do, sometimes not coming into play at all. (Ex: small heads.) It is good practice to section and cut the side caps in.

Pin or comb section I away. Comb side cap, above section E, straight down. Starting from the front of the head, lift comb and cut at angle shown, to and into the back section.

Sections F and G

Now we move to the opposite side of the head to sections F and G, following the same procedure as sections D and E. Don't forget the side cap.

Sections H, I, and J

Standing behind your client, start with the front of section H. Cut in one-quarter-inch to one-inch section strips. Cut back and into section A. (Be careful of crown area.)

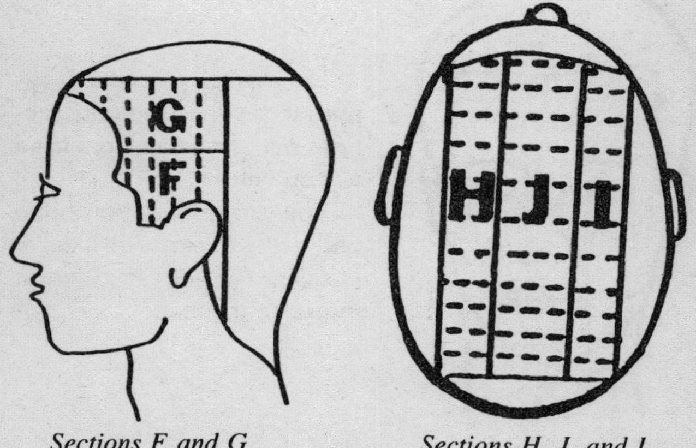

Sections F and G

Sections H, J, and I

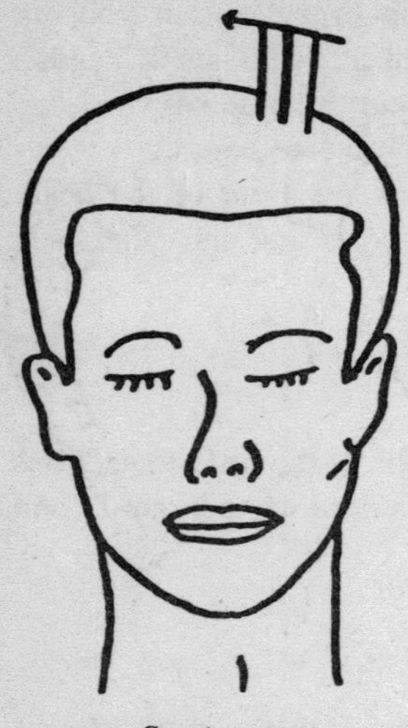

Section H

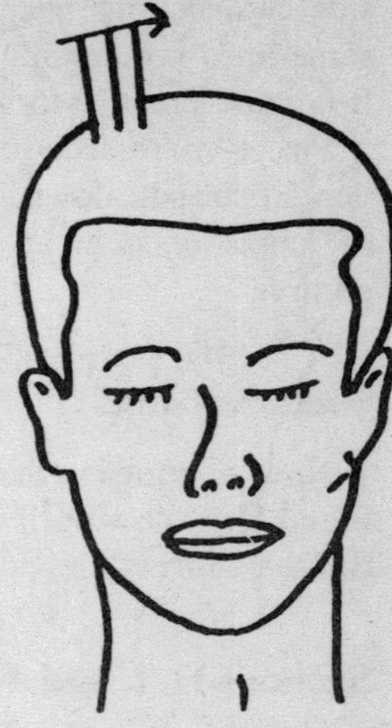

Section I

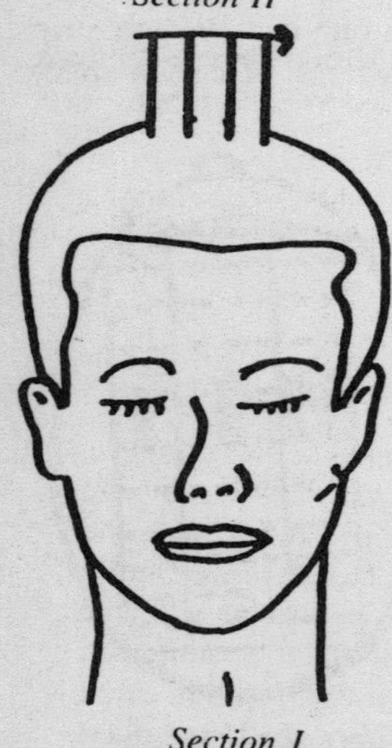

Section J

The same procedure applies to section I, holding sections out and away from head as you cut.

You can split section J into one or two parts—whatever is easier for you—and cut in the same manner.

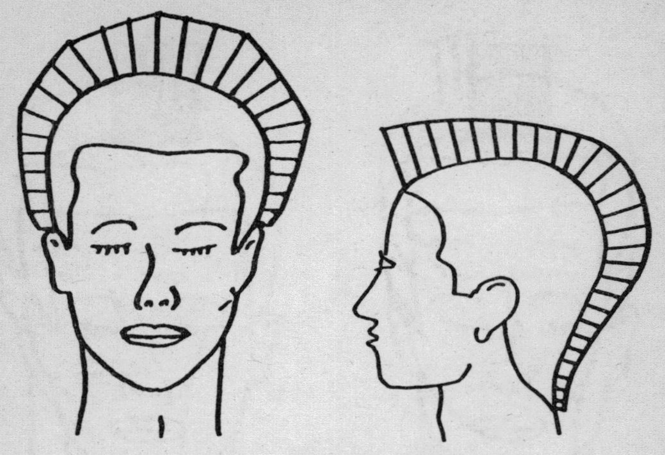

Check evenness of sections

Checking: Pick up the hair around the head where sections meet, making sure all sections blend into each other.

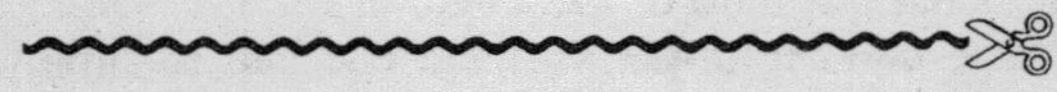

Thinning

Thinning is a procedure most layered haircuts can use. It takes the bulk out of the hair and makes it easier to comb and style. Thin hair more where it has bulk and less or not at all where it is not as bulky, being careful not to make it too thin. One or two strokes with the thinning shears at each section strip should be sufficient.

To thin layered haircuts, take your basic section strips, hold out at a ninety-degree angle from head, and make

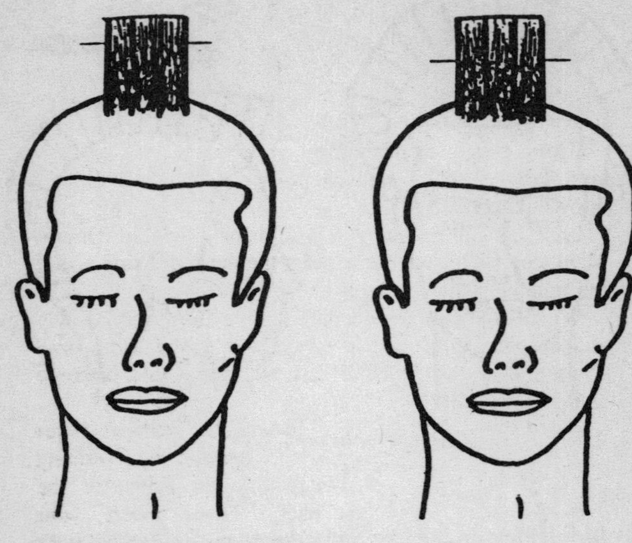

your cut about one-third of the length in toward roots.

For more thinning, make your cut one half to two-thirds in. This is good for wavy or curly hair.

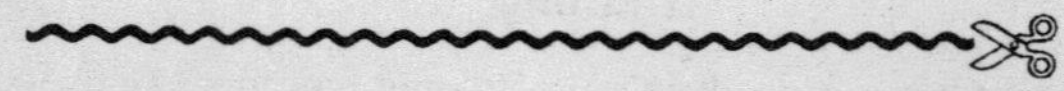

Scissors Over Comb Method

Short styles with a tapered look (going from very short to a longer length) require this method. You can only get so close picking the hair up with your fingers. To get closer, you must use scissors over comb.

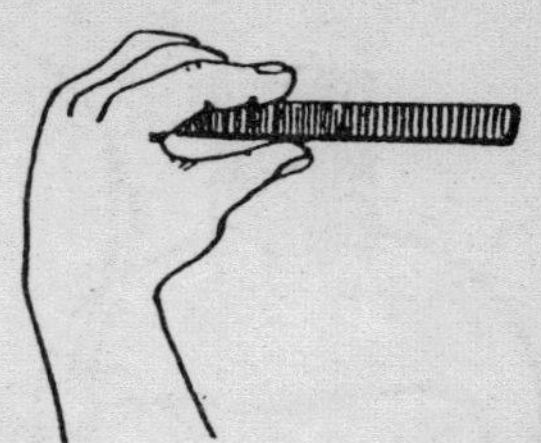

Hold comb with thumb and next two fingers, for most control and feel.

First, cut the hair as you would for a layered haircut. Then, cut as close at the nape of the neck and side, using the fingers.

When doing this procedure, move the comb slowly and continuously up and away, and at the same time continuously cut with the scissors, about two or three cuts a second.

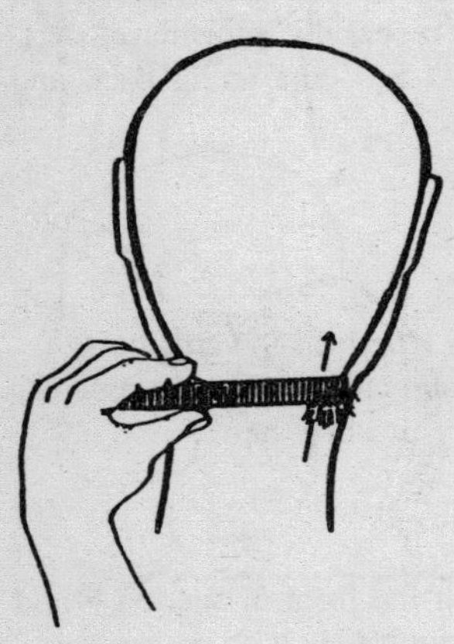

Start the scissors over comb method by combing hair straight down at the back. Then, insert your comb at the extreme bottom right of section C, picking up the hair out and away from the head only about one-eighth inch and make your first cut.

Your next cut will be just slightly higher but one-quarter inch away from the head.

The next cut will be slightly higher than the previous cut, about three-eighth inch out and away from the head, and so on, until you get a smooth cut blending into the higher elevations of the haircut.

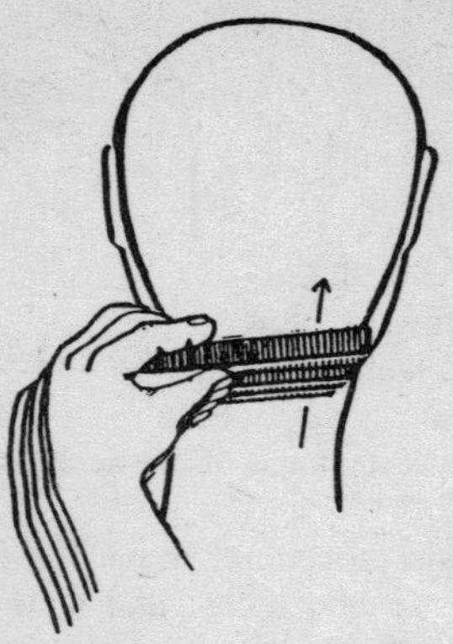

Move to the next part of section C and do the same thing. Continue this procedure all across section C.

Now go to section D and repeat this procedure, starting at the front of section D and continuing back and into section C.

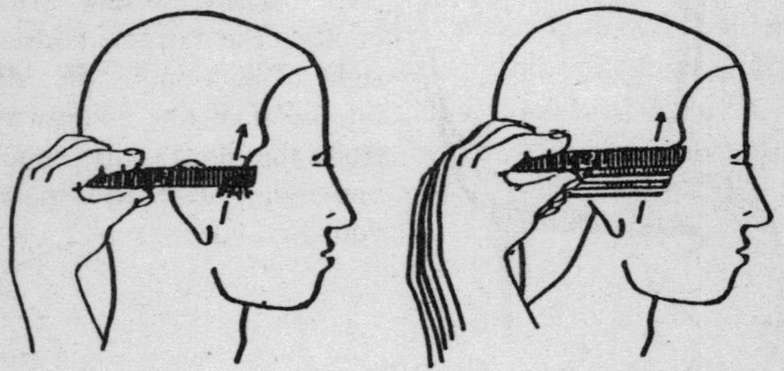

Go to section F, starting at the front of section F and continuing back and into section C.

When you are done with this procedure, you may find some steps in the hair. This can be somewhat corrected by taking your thinning shears, picking up the hair where the step is with your comb, and giving it a few cuts with the thinning shears until it is blended.

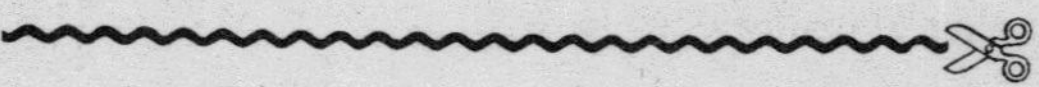

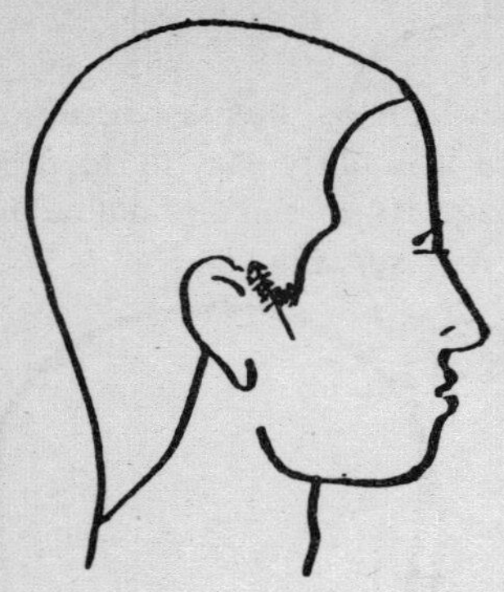

Cut sideburn design line

Sideburns

If your client is a male, you will want to trim his sideburns. Sideburns must be cut with the scissors over comb method. Cut most of the bulk away with scissors over comb and then cut the design line in as shown, making sure not to make the sideburn width too thin. Cut to desired length (light downstroke) with trimmer.

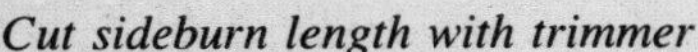

Cut sideburn length with trimmer

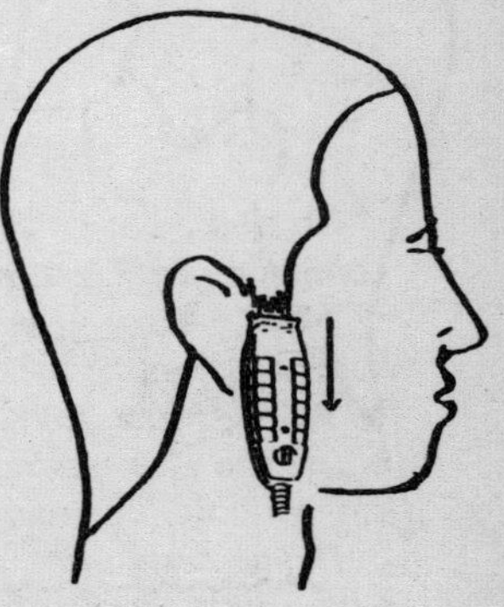

Finishing

On short to medium layered haircuts, this is where you get your professional look and it is fairly easy to do. You will need your trimmer (see page 10) to make or define the design line you created with your scissors.

Comb all the hair straight down in the back and sides. Starting from the neck, clean off straggly hairs on the neck with an upstroke, being careful not to go too high and into the nape area.

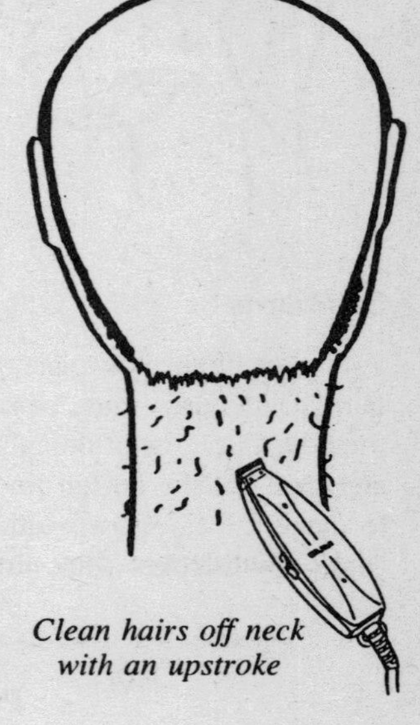

Clean hairs off neck with an upstroke

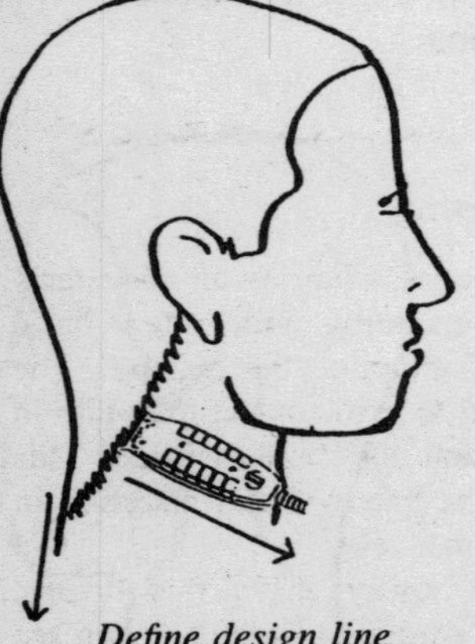

Define design line with a light downstroke

Next, comb hair at neck in design line direction, taking trimmer in a *light downstroke* and cutting a sharp line along back hair line. Brush clipped hairs away. Blow-dry and comb.

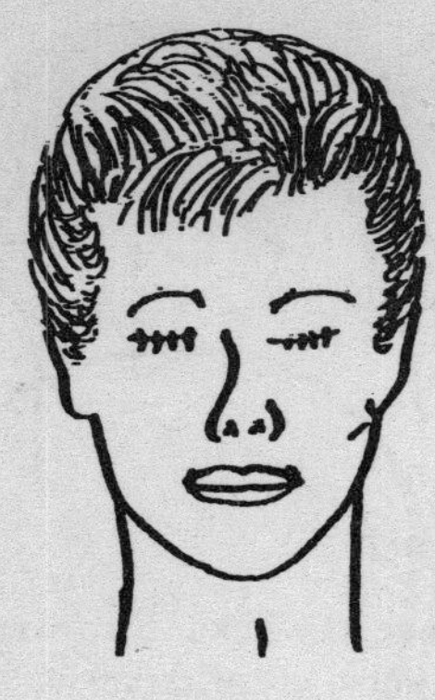

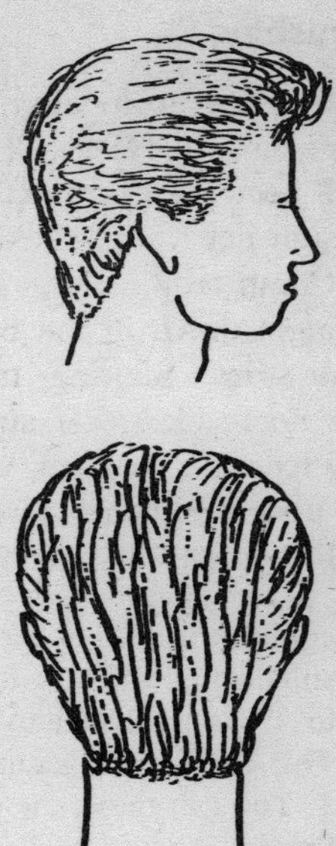

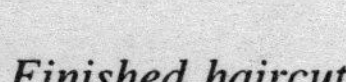

Finished haircut

Congratulations, you are done!

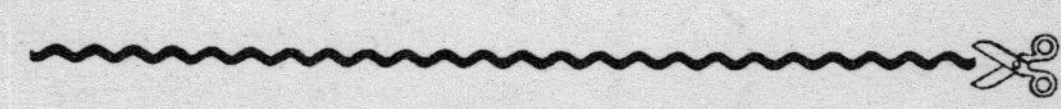

Parting

Finding the part in someone's hair is an easy task. Usually the part will fall naturally with a few basic movements. But first, let's examine the hairline. The ideal situation is for the hair to grow out of the scalp in a forward direction all along the front hairline. This gives you much leeway. The hair will fall naturally in a low part, high part, or center part.

Unfortunately, we don't always have this luxury. Look closely at your client's front hairline. You can see that not all hairlines are created equal. Some grow in

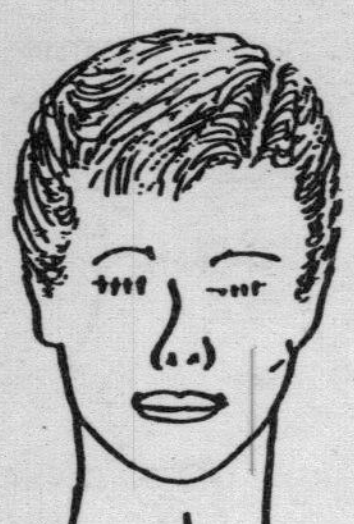
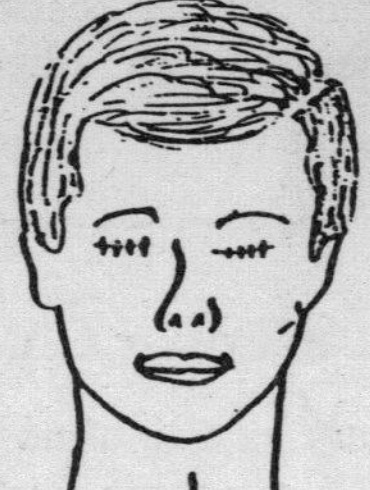
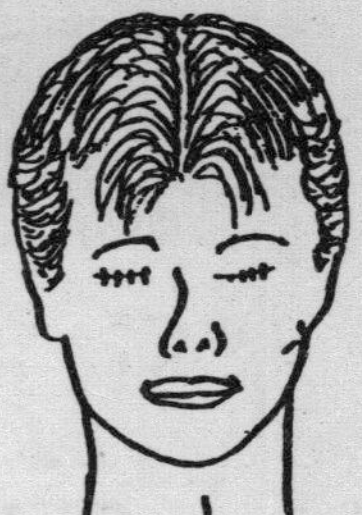

Typical parting

different directions and some have cowlicks. However, this basic procedure works on almost all of them.

After shampooing the hair, with your styling brush or comb, brush all of the hair straight back. The hair itself should find the part for you. It will split where it wants to. Coax the hair into the part with your brush or comb. This is the most natural area to part the hair.

You can move the part up or down as your style designates. Not all heads will react the same. Some will be more willing than others.

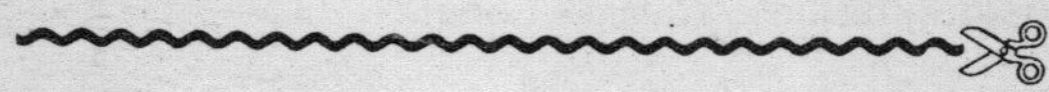

Correcting Mistakes

As a beginner, you will probably make some mistakes in your haircutting. Do not fear: Most mistakes can be corrected, or at least fixed to a point where you can't really notice them.

On most cuts, steps in the hair can be corrected by using your thinning shears. Pick up the area with your fingers or comb, depending on the length of the hair, and correct the step by blending with your thinning shears until the step disappears or lessens to a degree where it is not noticeable. Cutting the hair shorter beyond the mistake is another possibility, but if the mistake is too deep into the hair, a happy medium must be met.

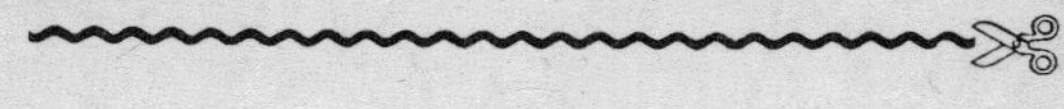

Clipper Cuts

Effects that are very hard or almost impossible to achieve with your scissor and comb are fairly easy to achieve with your clipper.

The Barber Taper

The barber taper is one clipper cut that takes a little practice. The barber taper goes from extremely short at the nape of the neck and sides, and gradually becomes longer and longer as it gets into the higher elevations of the cut.

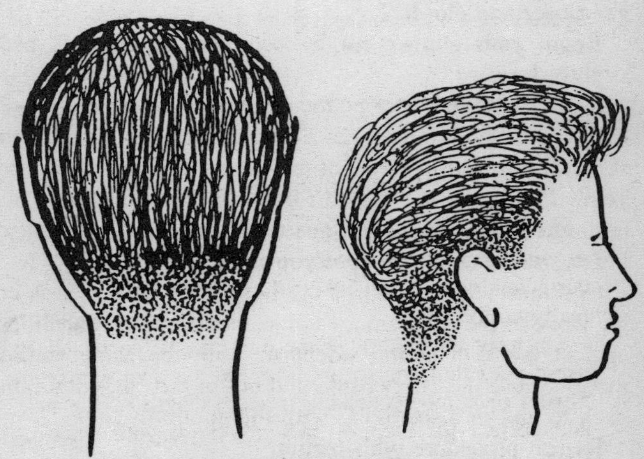

Barber taper

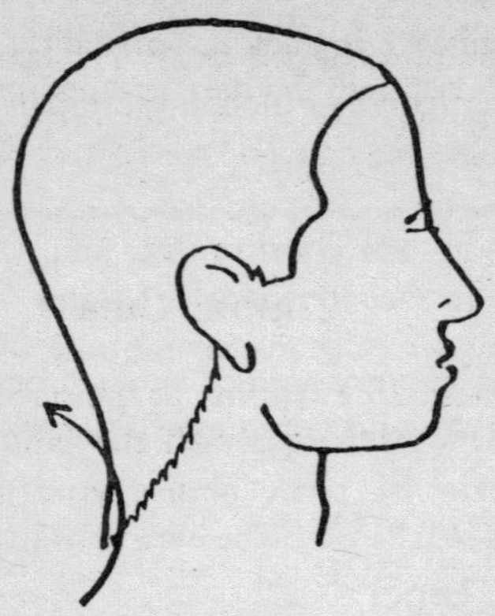

Start the barber taper cut at section C

Start with a large blade—a #2 size head is preferable and easier to use. The large head will enable you to stay farther from the scalp as you cut. Then you can switch blades to get closer and closer.

Begin your clipper cut by bending the patron's head slightly forward.

Next, start your cut at the bottom right of section C, below the natural hairline. Place the clipper against the skin, raise the clipper and, at the same time, curve it toward yourself out of the cut—sort of an arching motion. Total motion is about one-and-a-quarter to three inches, depending on how extreme a taper you prefer.

Continue left until all of the bottom of section C is cut in. Move to the sideburn area of section D. Place the clipper against the skin at the sideburn. With the same arching motion, raise the clipper into and out of the cut, continuing back to and into section C with this motion.

Repeat procedure with section F.

Now, give a normal layered haircut, blending section

strip by strip into clipped area. The scissors over comb method is a must when blending clipper cuts.

At this point, we can go one of two ways to finish the bottom.

The first is to take your trimmer and, with a downstroke, cut a design line at the nape area and sides of the neck. Don't go too high. Cut the design line as low as possible, but still maintain an even line at the nape.

The second way to finish off the bottom is to set your clipper with the #1 blade or use your trimmer. BE EXTREMELY CAREFUL. The wrong move here is hard to fix.

Use a very light arching upstroke along the bottom of sections C, D, and F, and just take the edge off. Then, cut in a design line at the nape and sides of the neck area with the trimmer.

Another option is the 000 blade, which is to be used after #1 and before the trimmer; but be very careful, the 000 is really close.

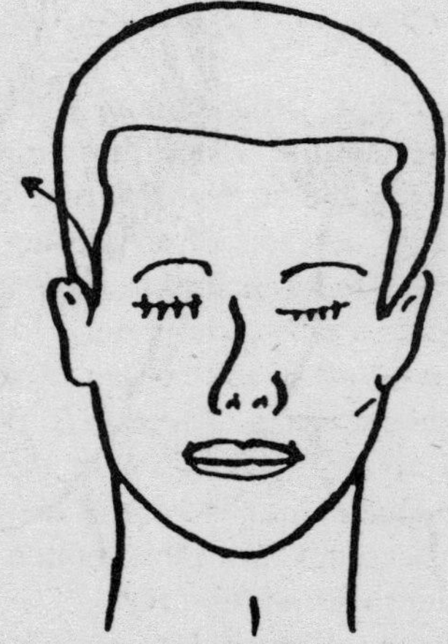

Clipping the sideburn area of section D

You may find a few spots in the tapered area that need blending. This can be done with scissors over comb *only*.

Insert your comb where hair is heavier, then directly below.

Make hair stand up by slightly twisting your comb into the scalp to make the very short hairs pick up.

Lift comb as you cut and, at the same time, bring it out and away from the head. Blend into shorter area. Be *extremely* careful not to cut too deep. Do a little at a time and it will blend.

The Ridge Cut Buzz Cut

This cut is very striking, and it's popular with the younger set of males and females. There are many variations. The most popular two are the one-length ridge cut

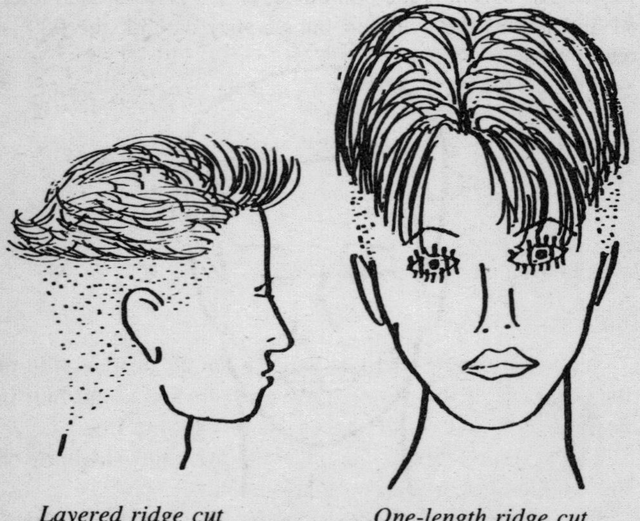

Layered ridge cut *One-length ridge cut*

and the layered ridge cut. This haircut has two design lines; one at the extreme bottom and one that is one to two inches or more up from the bottom.

The one-length ridge cut must have enough length on the top to reach the ridge.

Section long hair away, leaving sections C, D, and F exposed.

Start by using your #2 blade or adjustment. If you feel you want it closer, you can always cut tighter later.

Cut all around sections C, D, and F by putting the blade against the skin and raising it flat to the scalp, up about one-and-a-half to three-and-a-half inches, depending on the look you prefer.

Comb sections B, E, and F down over buzzed area. With your scissors, cut the first design line from the front of section E, around and into section B, and into and to the end of section F. This design line must hang over the buzzed area by at least a half inch.

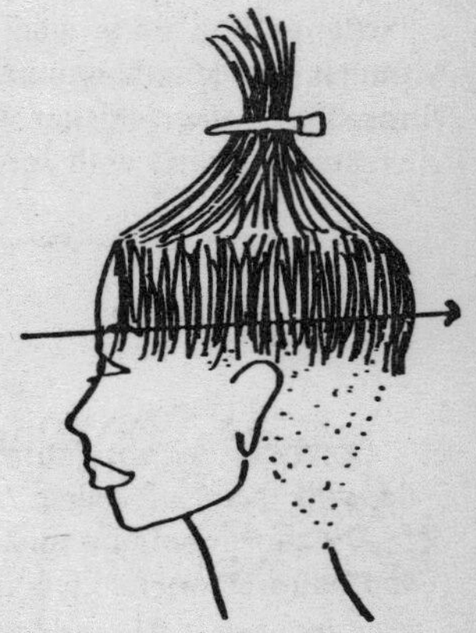

The design line must hang over the buzzed area

With this cut, the hair is usually parted on one side or the other, or in the center. Find the part and comb hair in desired style and cut off excess at first design line.

Cut a second design line at nape area and sideburn on the male and nape area on the female.

For a layered ridge cut, follow exactly the same procedure as a one-length ridge cut, but in this case, after the ridge is cut in, proceed with the basic cut, layering the hair.

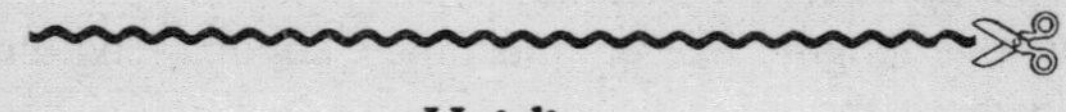

Hairlines

Hairlines are as different as hairstyles. There are many to contend with. Sometimes you have to create one because the hair just is not there or there is so much hair that you have to define where the hairline is. Usually, it is clearly visible.

Examine the neck area and around the ears carefully before cutting. You can see where the natural hairline is thicker and where the hair thins out, kind of hiding in the growth. This is where you cut your design line in on shorter length haircuts. If the hair is very thin or missing, leave it thicker when you do your basic cut and create a hairline with scissors or trimmer.

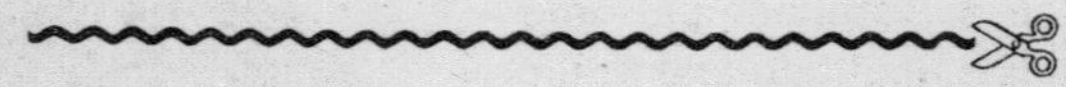

Cowlicks

Cowlicks are a nightmare—unless you know what to do with them, of course.

The most common mistake many barbers, hairstylists, and hairdressers make is in the crown area, which is the area located at the top back, left, or right portion of the head. The hair usually will grow in a circle. If this area is cut too short, it most likely will stand up. Unless you want this look, it will not do justice to your haircut.

Examine the growth pattern of the hair. The crown is usually on the left or right side of the head. If the hairstyle you are doing requires a part, part the hair from the crown side over to the opposite side of the head and it will lie down nicely. Parting it on the opposite side of the crown will make the hair stand up because you are pushing the hair against the growth pattern. You can be less concerned with the crown area on hairstyles that are combed back. When in doubt, leave this area a little longer at first, then cut a little at a time. When you see the area start to perk up a bit, you have cut enough. It is a good idea to use the thinning shears to cut this area since they cut just a portion of the hair. They are a little more forgiving. It will take longer, but it will lessen mistakes.

Cowlicks at the front hairline are a little more difficult to deal with. The general agreement is to leave this area a little longer so it will not stand up. Try to incorporate it into your hairstyle. On hair combed back, utilize the front cowlick to enhance your style for a carefree look, or split the cowlick into combed back or parted hair.

Double crown cowlicks or double front cowlicks are usually aided by extra length.

Quick Step Guide

1. Shampoo hair, towel dry, but leave hair damp.
2. Section, or imagine where sections should be.
3. Cut in section strips, six to ten a section (section strips should be approximately a quarter inch to one inch wide and two inches to three inches long).
4. *Section A:* Start with back right of section A. Lift hair out and away from head to cut (ninety-degree rule). Section and cut across all of section A.
5. *Section B:* Cut from right to left. Pick up a bit of section A for length comparison with each section strip. Cut on an angle shorter at bottom, longer at top.
6. *Section C:* Cut right to left. Blend with section B and angle as desired for length at bottom.

7. Cut design line in at neck area.
8. *Section D:* Comb away section E, cut section D from front to back into B and C, angling as desired for length at side.
9. Comb section D straight down and cut design line at length desired. Blend with neck area design line.
10. *Section E:* Cut to and into sections A and B.
11. *Side Cap:* Section and cut to and into the back section.
12. *Sections F and G:* Same procedure as D and E and side cap.
13. *Sections H, I, and J:* Stand behind client. Cut section H from front to back, followed by section I, then section J.
14. Blend all sections.
15. Thin hair as needed.
16. Finish with trimmer.

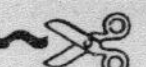 5

Medium and Long Layered Haircuts

Cutting the Front

Here are a few different ways to even the front.

The easiest way is to comb the hair straight down and cut it evenly all across. This method will leave the underneath hair short and the outer hair long. This is fine for a bang-style haircut. However, this gives us little leeway with the final design on side parts and styles that are brushed back.

If the hair seems too long at the front—and to ensure the proper length for the bottom front hair—the correct way to cut is as follows (after the hair is cut using the ninety-degree rule):

Comb the bang area forward and, in three or four sections, pull the hair as far forward as it can go. Cut the front evenly all across.

On side-parted hair, leave enough length for the hair to hold itself when brushed to the side.

Beveling

On hair that is longer (longer layered cuts or one length cuts), it is a good idea to bevel the nape area. Beveling leaves the outer portion of the hair slightly longer. This bit of extra length will create a natural tendency to curve under and give more control to this area.

Before you cut the back design line, tilt the head forward toward the chest. Then, cut in the design line, holding the hair as close to the neck as possible.

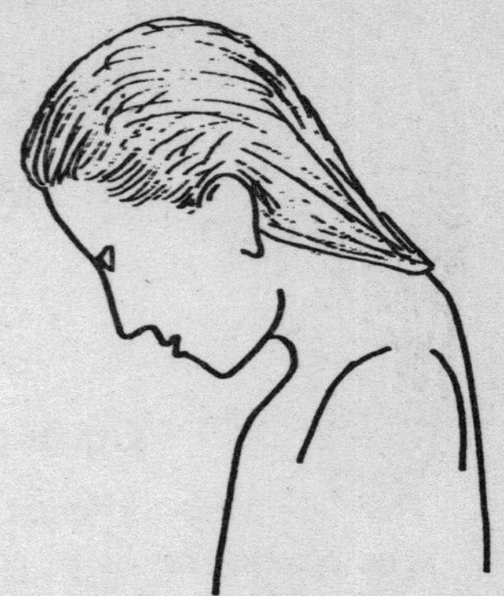

Tilt the head forward

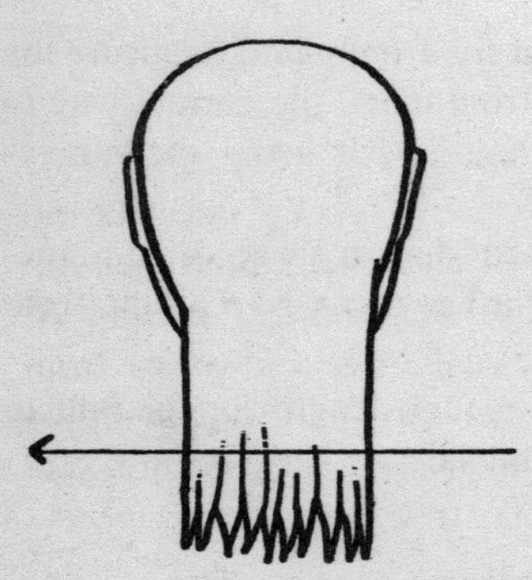

Cut in the design line

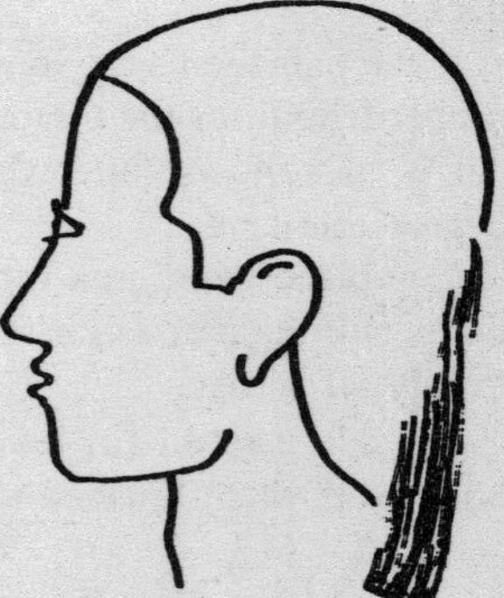

Beveled design line

Longer Layers

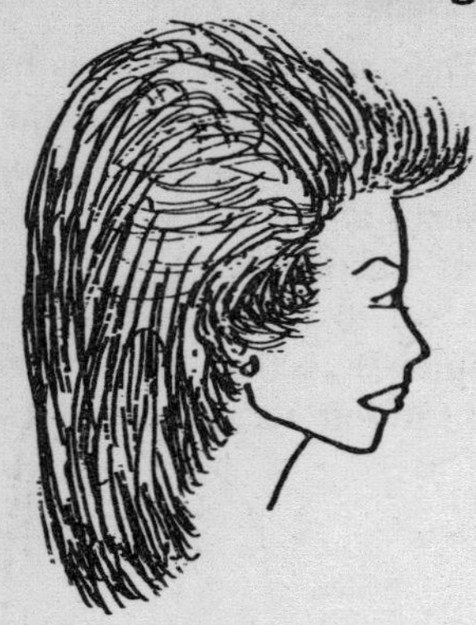

Medium to long layered hair is cut basically the same as short to medium layered haircuts. Sections are cut using the section-section-strip method, but layers are left longer and angles are more extreme.

Layers are longer and angles are more extreme

Follow the sectioning of the basic short to medium cut, but adjust the length and angles of the different sections to fit the cut and style you want to finish with.

Section strips will still be cut six to ten a section, but the length will be longer (approximately three inches to six inches long).

Section A

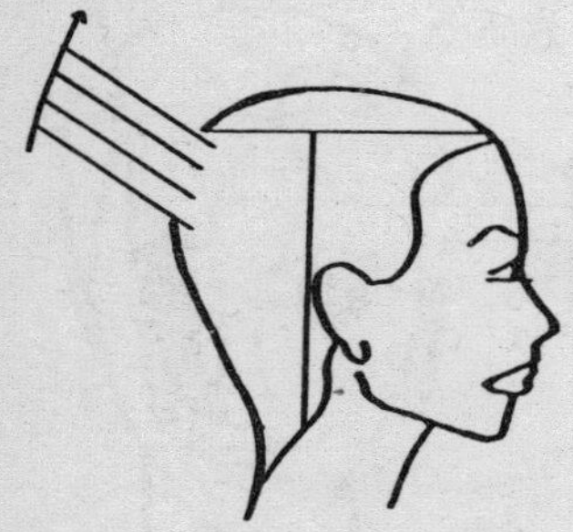

Comb or clip side and top sections away. Starting with the back right of section A, lift hair out and away from head and hold diagonally as shown, and cut your first section strip.

Cut your first section strip

Continue to cut section strips from right to left across all of section A.

Section B

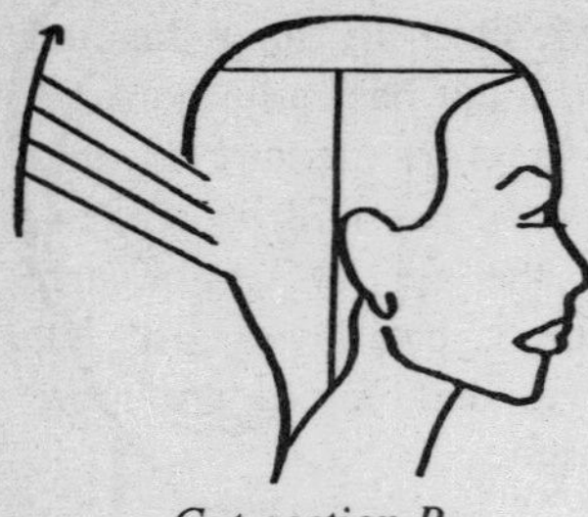
Cut section B

The same angle applies to section B. Starting from the right of section B, lift section B strips at this extreme angle using section A as a guide and cut to match angle. Cut section B section strips from right to left across all of section B.

Section C

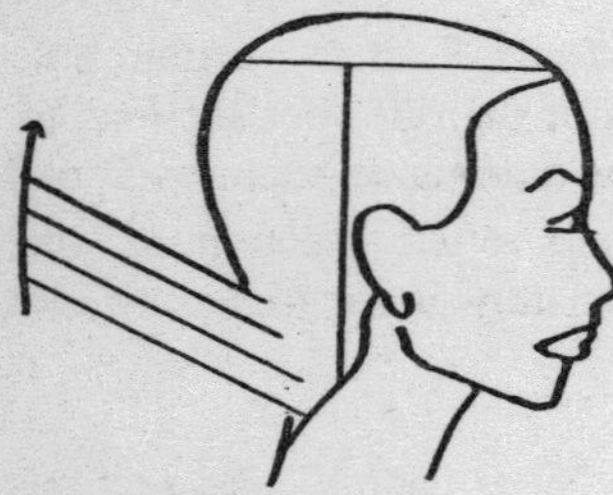
Cut section C

Section C is cut at the same angle as sections A and B. This extreme angle will leave length at the bottom for the hair to lie properly for a longer look.

Section D

Section away section E and above. Comb section D down, then cut section D in usual section-strip method, regulating length with fingers. Cut section D to and into sections B and C.

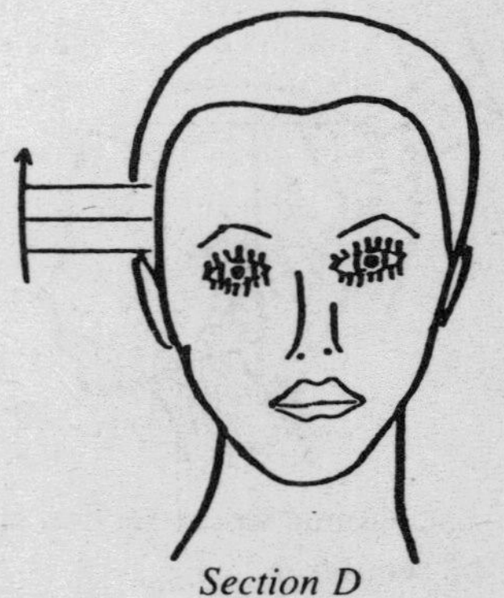
Section D

Section E

Next, comb section E down over section D. Cut section E in section strips to and into sections A and B. Comb hair forward at front of sections D and E and trim excess.

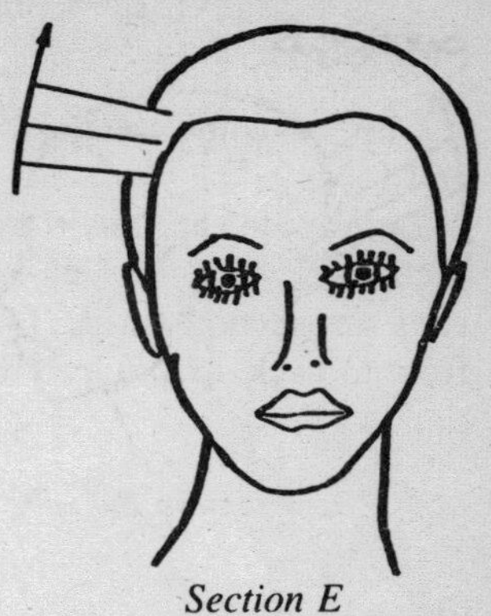

Section E

Sections F and G

Cut sections F and G in same manner as sections D and E.

Design Line

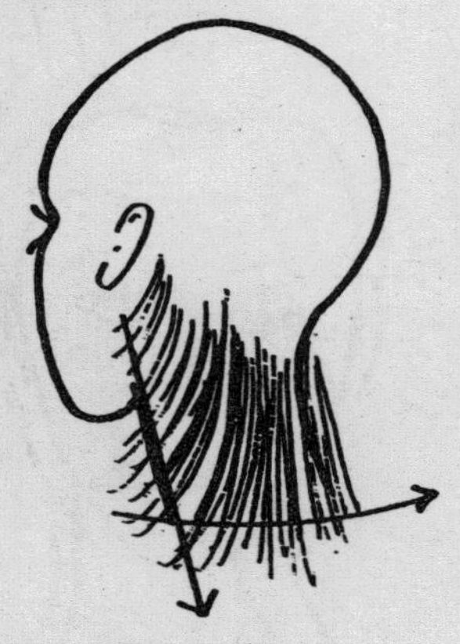

Design line

Next, comb all sections previously cut down, curving the sides of the nape area in, cut design line at desired length along the bottom perimeter. When cutting the bottom, tilt the head forward to bevel.

Side Caps

Clip or comb sections H and I away.

Comb side caps down over sections E and F. Cut side caps in section strips from front to back, to and into section A.

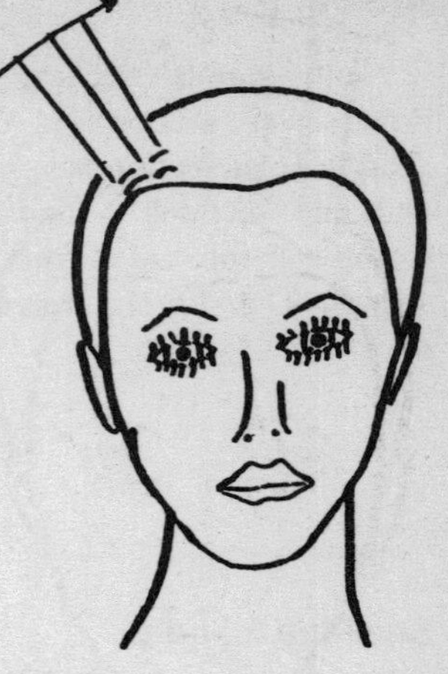

Side Caps

Sections H, I, and J

Standing behind your client, start with the front of section H. Cut in a quarter inch- to one inch-wide section strips. Cut back and into section A. (Be careful of crown area.)

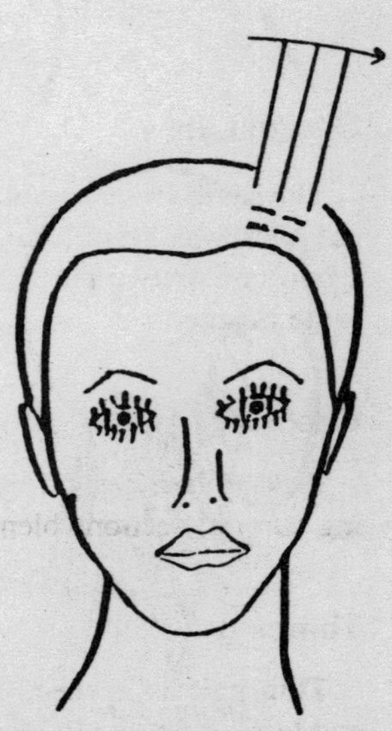

Section H

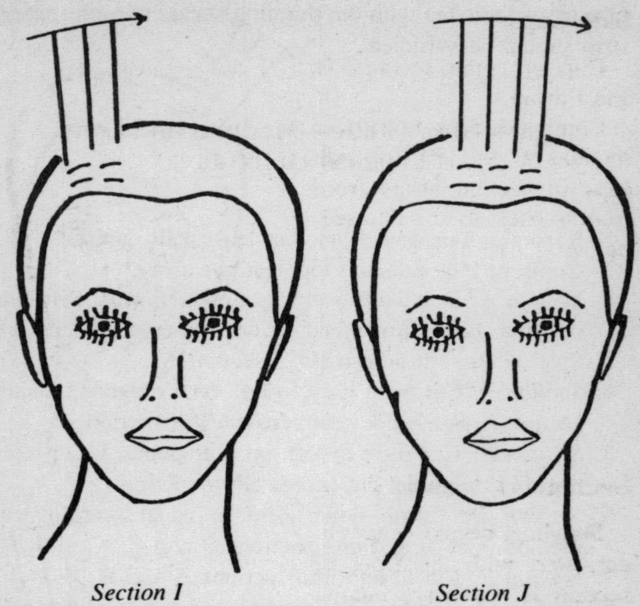

Section I　　*Section J*

The same procedure applies to section I, holding sections out and away from head as you cut. You can split section J into one or two parts, whatever is easier for you. Cut in same manner.

Checking

Pick up hair around the head where sections meet, making sure all sections blend into each other.

Thinning

Thin hair as needed. Thin hair more where it has bulk and less, or not at all, where it is less bulky. Do not overdo.

One or two strokes with the thinning shears at each section strip should be sufficient.

Quick Step Guide—Medium and Long Layered Haircuts

1. Shampoo hair, towel dry, but leave hair damp.
2. Comb or clip side and top sections away.
3. *Section A:* Start with back right of section A. Lift hair out and away from head to cut (ninety-degree rule). Section and cut across all of section A.
4. *Section B:* Cut from right to left, on a diagonal. Using section A as a guide, cut across all of section B.
5. *Section C:* Cut right to left, on a diagonal. Using section B as a guide, cut across all of section C.
6. *Section D:* Comb down. Cut in usual section-strip method. Cut to and into sections B and C.
7. *Section E:* Cut to and into sections A and B.
8. *Sections F and G:* Cut in same manner as sections D and E.
9. Comb down all sections previously cut and cut design line.
10. Side caps.
11. *Sections H, I, and J:* Stand behind client. Cut section H from front to back, followed by section I, then section J.
12. Blend and check all sections.
13. Thin hair as needed. Finish with trimmer if necessary.

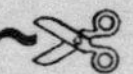

Feathering

Feathering hair is just what it sounds like—to make the hair lighter in weight. Usually, it's done on bangs or back nape area to eliminate a heavy line in these places.

Bangs

To feather bangs, cut in the bangs as you normally would (see "Adding Bangs" on page 58).

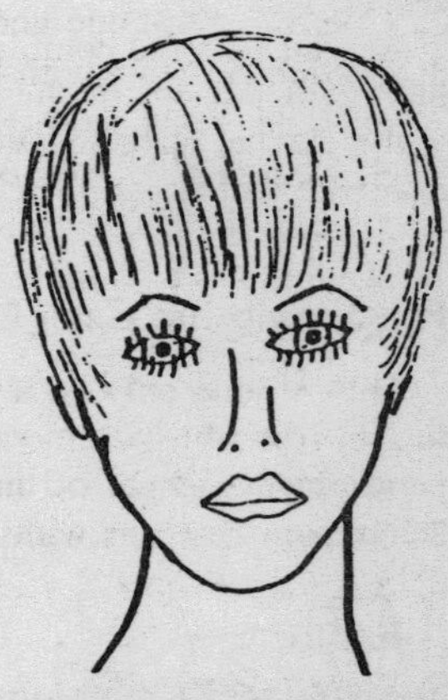

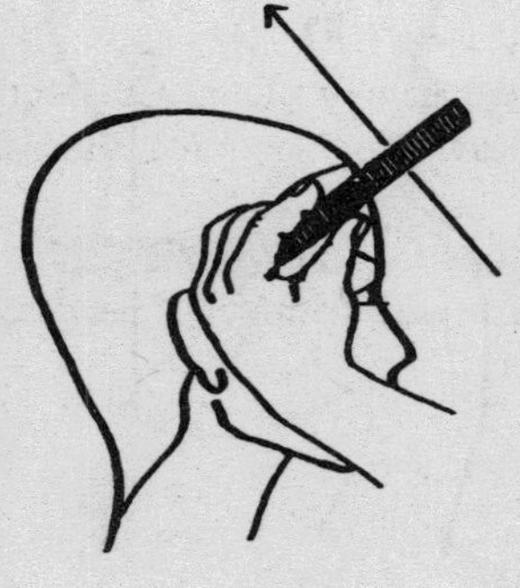

Standing in front of the client, use the comb to pick up a section of hair about one and a half inches wide on the right side of the bang area. At the same time, use your thinning shear to cut scissors over comb method at the angle shown, making sure you hold the hair out and away from the head as you cut.

As your comb slowly moves through the angled movement, cut with your thinning shears continuously (two to three cuts per second) throughout the full movement from beginning to end.

Cut in from the extreme ends about a half inch to three quarters of an inch for light feathering, one inch to three inches for heavy feathering.

Now move left to the next one and a half inch section of the bang area and repeat the process until the bang section is complete.

As you pass the comb through the angle, the bottom hairs will fall out of the cut. Repeating the procedure will make the feathered area lighter and lighter until the desired effect is achieved.

Feathering the Back Nape Area

This is done only on layered haircuts. However, cutting in from the extreme ends is a judgment call. It depends on the length of the hair of that area. The same technique is used as with the bangs.

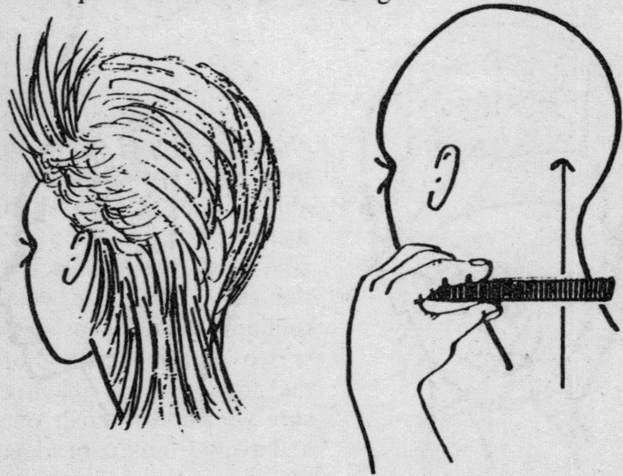

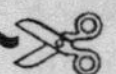

Sectioning Long, One-Length Hair

Before you begin to cut long, one-length hair, the hair above the section or sections you are cutting must be clipped out of the way so as not to conflict with the section to be cut.

Start with the back top right of the head. Section the back as shown.

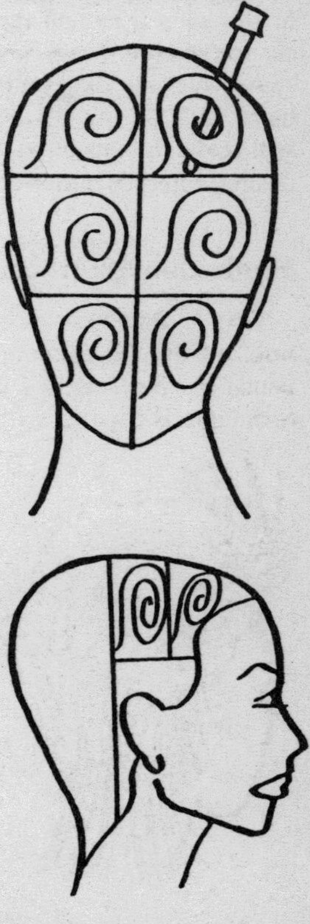

Section the back of long hair with clips

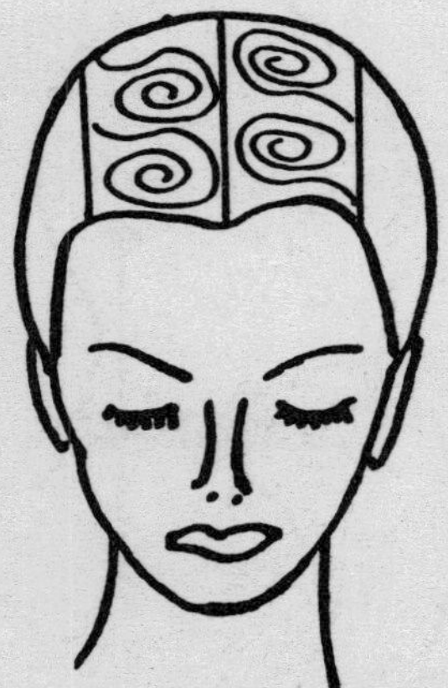

Section top of long hair

Section sides of long hair

Each section should be held out and away from the head at the bitter end, twisted two or three times, then placed back to the head, and the clip inserted.

This ensures that these sections will not get in your way as you proceed with your cut.

Section top and sides as shown.

As you proceed with the cut, unclip and drop the hair section by section, until the cut is complete.

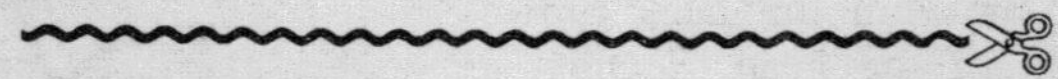

6

Long, One-Length Hair

Long, one-length hair is cut differently than layered hair. The sectioning will vary, depending on the cut you give.

To be a one-length cut, all hair on the head must be long enough to reach the design line, excluding the bang area. Some advanced cuts are exceptions to this general rule.

This cut can be given on many different lengths, including extra long hair, and can be cut with a center or side part.

So as not to confuse you with the sectioning for layered haircuts, we will use numbers instead of letters for the different sections of the one-length cut.

Let's start with a one-length blunt cut with a center part, with instructions in parenthesis for a side-parted cut.

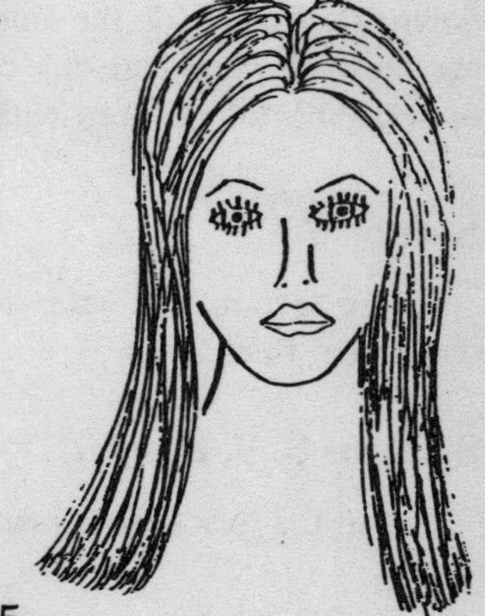

One-length blunt cut with a center part

Section 1

Separate and clip away all sections except section 1. Comb section 1 straight down and cut the design line across section 1 at the desired length.

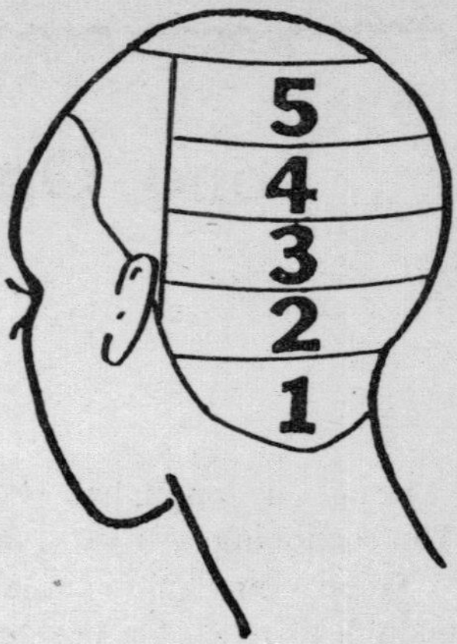

Section 2

Comb section 2 down and over section 1 and cut even with the design line.

Sections 3, 4, and 5

Cut in the exact same manner as above.

Back sections for long, one-length hair

Section 6

Clip away sections 7 to 10. Comb section 6 straight down. Depending on the angle you prefer (different angles are shown for comparison), cut a design line from the front of section 6 to and even with the back section design line.

Section 7

Comb section 7 down over section 6 and cut even with the design line.

Sections 8, 9, and 10

Cut in the exact same manner as above.

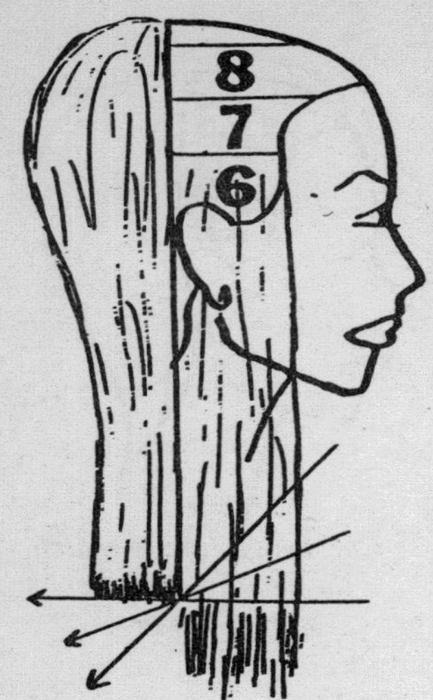

Section 6 can be cut at different angles

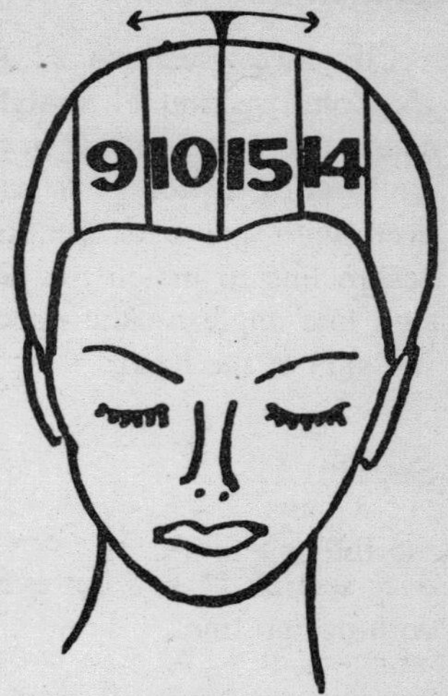

Cut these sections the same as the side sections

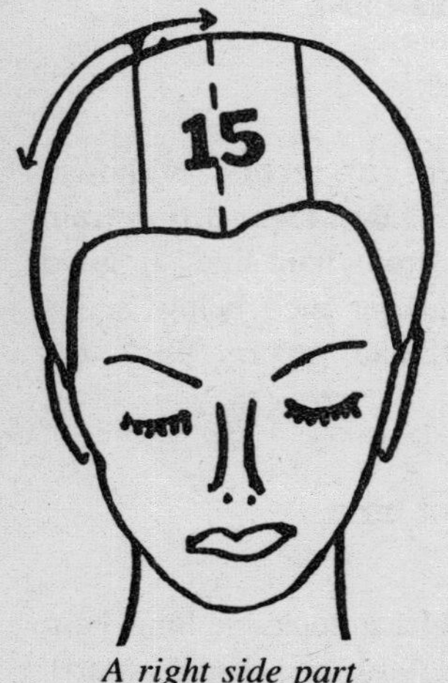

A right side part

(If you prefer a side part, regulate the sectioning to conform. For instance, for a right side part, sections 8 and 9 should be the last sections combed down and cut in on the right side. When on the left side, section 15 should be extended to compensate. For a left side part, extend section 10 over to the left side part area and sections 13 and 14 should be the last sections combed down and cut.)

Section 11

Clip away sections 12 to 15. Comb section 11 straight down. Cut a design line from the front of section 11 to and even with the back section design line to match the design line angle on the opposite side of the head.

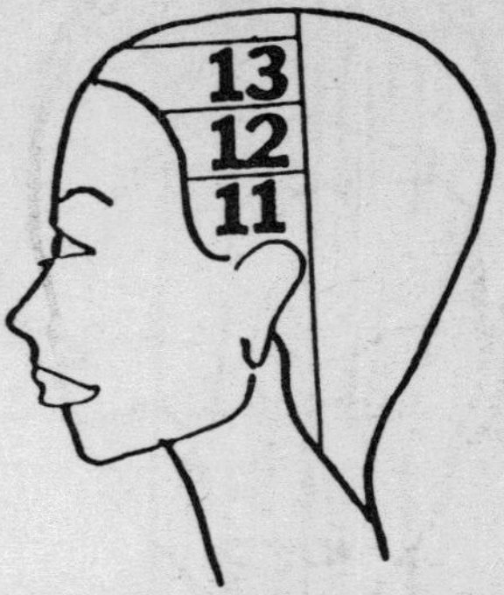

Cut design line to match the one on the other side of the head

Section 12

Comb section 12 down over section 11 and cut even with design line.

Sections 13, 14, and 15

Cut in the exact same manner as above.

Adding Bangs

To add bangs to your one-length cut, section as shown, taking care not to section too far back. Make section from two inches to four inches from front hair line. A good length for bangs is between a quarter inch below and a quarter inch above eyebrows. (If hair is very thick, cut bangs in two sections.)

Feathering the Sides and Front on a One-Length Haircut

To feather and get that swept-back look on long hair, after completing a one-length cut (with or without a part),

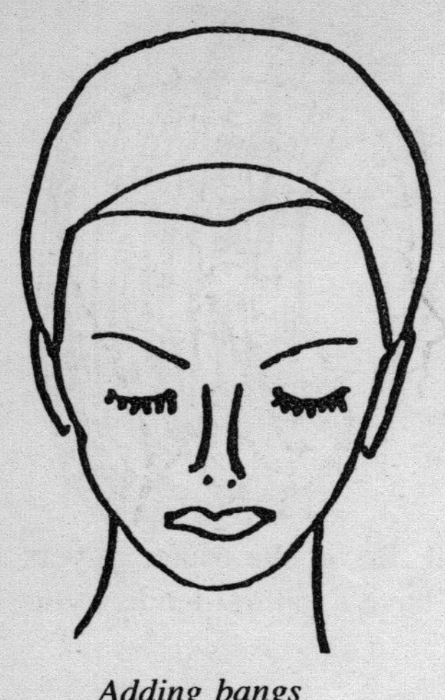

Adding bangs

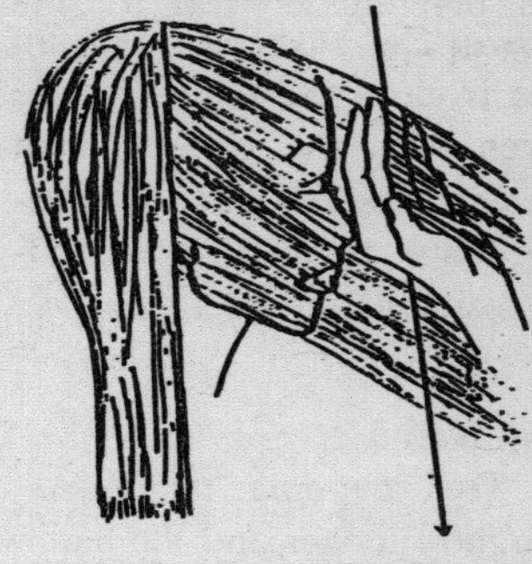

Feathering the sides and front on a one-length haircut

comb the front perimeter forward and cut at an angle shown on both sides of the head. Then, pick up the front bang section and cut section strips from two inches to four inches back from the hairline. Comb all sections that you just cut forward and blend front and side sections. Blow-dry back with center or side part.

Curling Under on a One-Length Haircut

The cupping effect at the design line is very attractive and gives a natural look. We can give this cut with or without bangs, or with the feathered look, as previously described. However, on extremely long hair (into the client's back area), this cut is not advised.

This will be a curling under, one-length cut with a center part, with instructions in parentheses for a side parted cut.

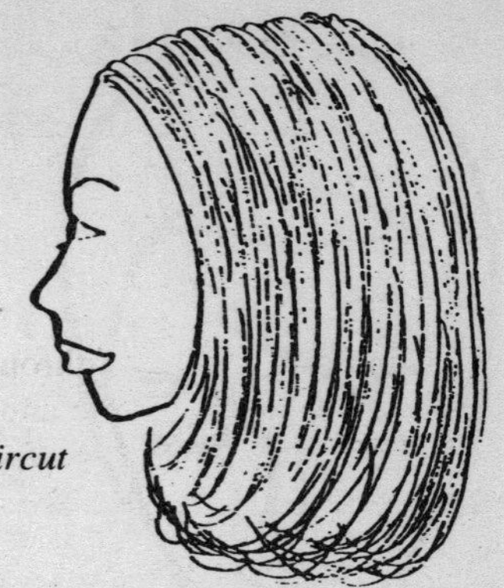

A curling under one-length haircut

This cupping technique will leave the outer layers slightly longer and the hair will have a natural tendency to curl under.

Section 1

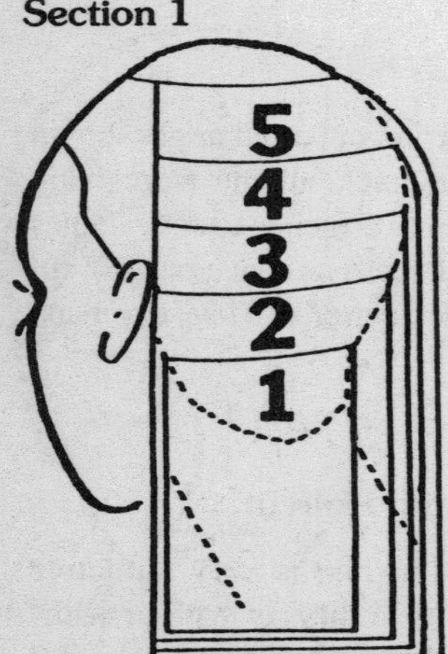

Section and clip away all sections, except section 1. Comb section 1 straight down and cut a design line approximately a half inch shorter than the final length desired.

Section 2

Comb section 2 down over section 1 and cut section 2 an eighth inch longer than section 1's design line.

Cut the design line for section 1 shorter than the final length desired

Sections 3, 4, and 5

These sections are each left an eighth inch longer than the previous section.

Section 6

Clip away sections 7 through 10. Comb section 6 straight down. Depending on the angle you prefer, cut a design line from the front of section 6 to, but a half inch shorter than, the back section design line.

Section 7

Comb section 7 down over section 6 and cut an eighth inch longer than section 6's design line.

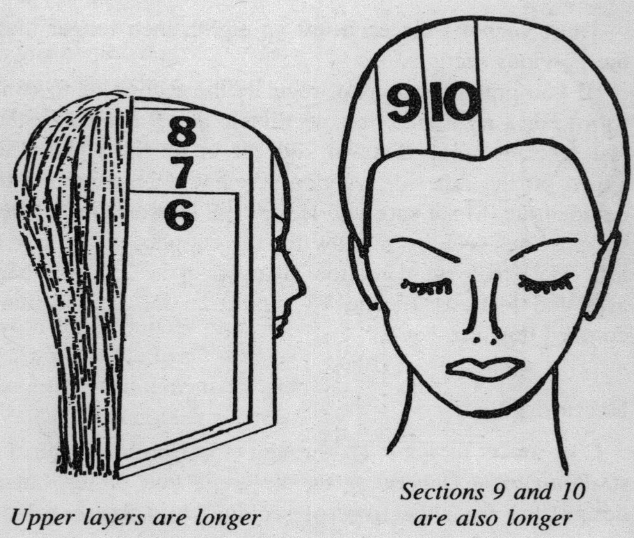

Upper layers are longer

Sections 9 and 10 are also longer

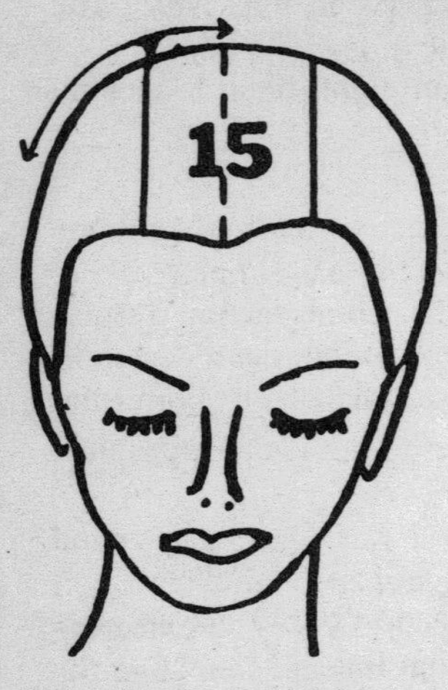

A right side part

Sections 8, 9, and 10

These sections are each left an eighth inch longer than the previous sections.

(If you prefer a side part, regulate the sectioning to conform. For a right side part, sections 8 and 9 should be the last sections combed down and cut in on the right side. When on the left side, section 15 should be extended to compensate. Make sure you leave each section longer than the previous section to allow for the cupping effect. For a left side part, extend section 10 over to the left side part area and sections 13 and 14 should be the last sections combed down to cut.)

Section 11

Clip away sections 12 through 15. Comb section 11 straight down. Depending on the angle you prefer, cut a design line from the front of section 11 to, but one half inch shorter than, the back section design line. *Note:* The design line should be even on both sides.

Section 12

Comb section 12 down over section 11 and cut one eighth inch longer than the section 11 design line.

Sections 13, 14, and 15

These sections are each left one eighth inch longer than the previous section.

Blow-dry with a curling-under motion, using a round styling brush or a curling iron for stubborn hair.

Also see "Adding Bangs" on page 58 and "Feathering the Sides and Front of a One-Length Haircut" on page 58.

Blow-Drying

Blow-drying hair is not only just to get the moisture out, blow-drying can create volume in flat areas or flatten puffy ones. It can give body to the hair for style manageability. It can revive a tired looking haircut to a cut that is full and bounces. Blow-drying is a setting process. For best results, the hair must be freshly shampooed.

Before you begin to blow-dry, towel dry the hair and leave it damp. Gel, mousse, etc. is optional.

Vigorously move your fingers followed by the blow-dryer throughout the head to get most of the moisture out.

Caution: Never hold the blower closer to the hair than four inches. Be careful not to burn the hair when drying. When using a heat and cool method, hold the blower about four inches away for no more than two seconds.

Heat and Cool

The hair will become pliable when heat is applied. It will harden when moisture is taken away and it is allowed to cool. The hair does not react to the blower until 95 percent of the moisture is gone. Use your nylon styling brush for the blow-out.

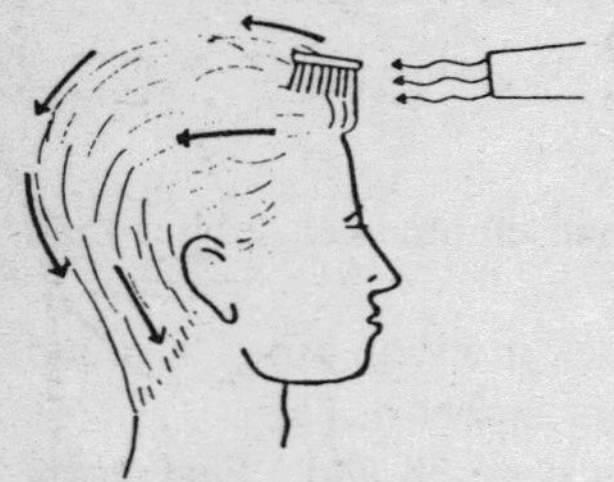

Heat and cool

In a simple blow-dry technique, the direction of the blow-dryer should follow the direction of the brush, and the brush should follow the direction of the style.

Heat, Twist, and Cool

Heat, twist, and cool in section strips. As you blow-dry the hair, in the areas where you need more volume, insert your brush into the hair and down to the scalp. Slightly twist the brush to lift the hair (the more you twist, the more lift you will get). Heat with the blower about four inches away for a few seconds, remove heat, let cool for about three to five seconds, and remove the brush. The hair will retain the

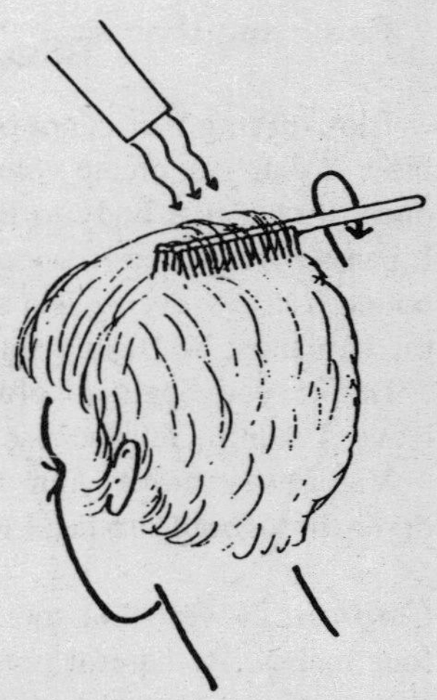

Heat, twist, and cool

lift. Heat, twist, and cool the areas that need volume, then brush out for style.

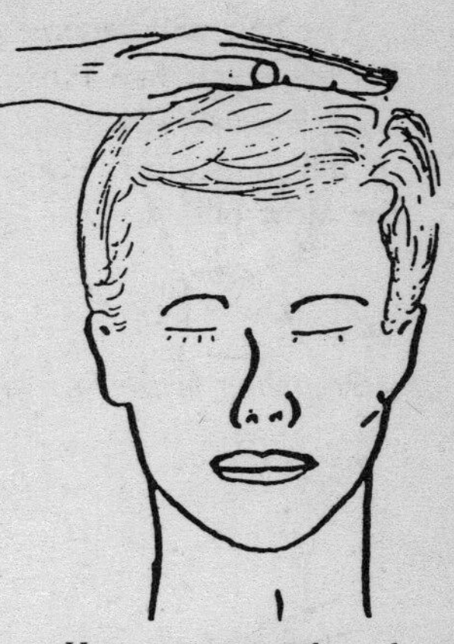

Heat, press, and cool

Heat, Press, and Cool

If you have a high spot in the hairstyle, a simple way to flatten it is to heat with the blow-dryer, remove the heat, and press down on the high area until it is cool.

Removing Waves

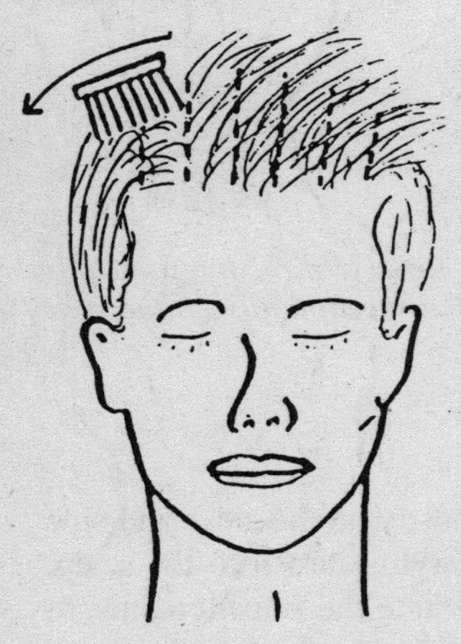

Removing waves

Hair gel or mousse, etc., is an effective aid on wavy hair. Blow-dry the opposite way of the finished style. Dry until about 95 percent of the moisture is removed and then brush back in section strips, followed by the blower, to desired style.

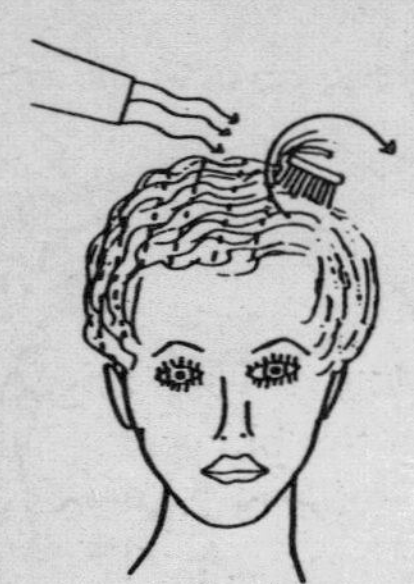

Insert styling brush to scalp

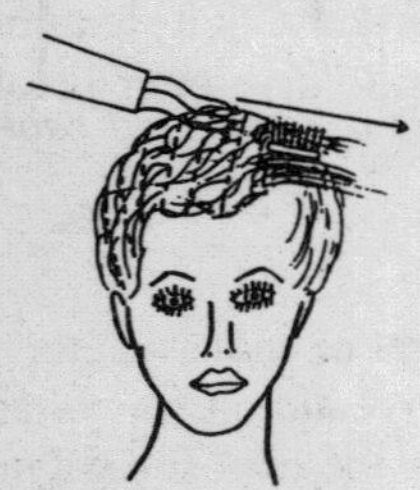

Slightly twist brush, rotate counter to the wave, and pull in the opposite direction to the wave

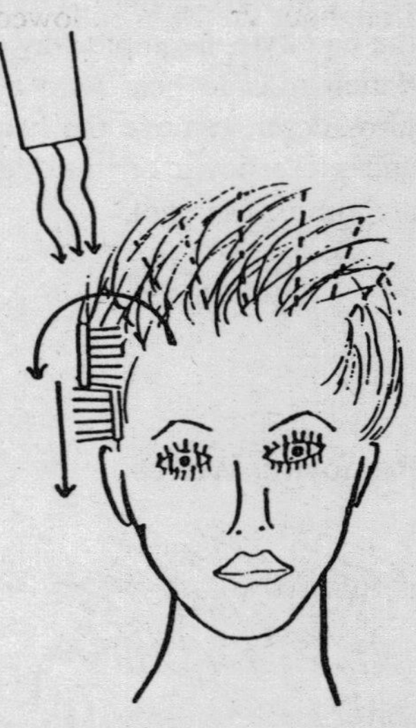

Reverse direction to blend hair section in with the style

Stretch

To remove stubborn waves, mostly on the sides and side parted styles, insert your nylon styling brush to the scalp. Slightly twist to grab the hair, rotate the brush counter to the wave, and pull in the opposite direction of the wave, section strip by section strip, again removing 95 percent of the moisture. When the section is complete, reverse the action until blended with the style.

Blowing Out Long Hair

On longer layered styles, vigorously move your fingers throughout the head followed closely by the blower.

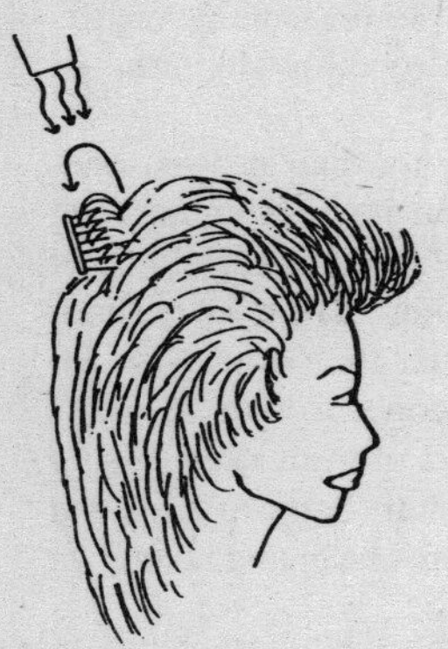
Blowing out long layered hair

A vent type brush works best for the next step. By section strip, insert the brush into the hair. Use a twisting motion to lift the hair, blow, hold a second and let go. This will add body and texture. Repeat until dry, then brush into the desired style.

Long, One-Length Hair

Dry using a twist and pull method to add body. Clip away the sides and top. Working with the back, clip away the top three quarters of the hair and blow dry underneath first. When dry, drop a second section down over the first and blow dry, then a third section, and a fourth, if necessary. Repeat this procedure on the sides and top.

Any of the blow-dry methods described here can be mixed and matched. Be creative. Try different methods on different heads. You will soon see what works best and where.

Cutting the Hair for Perm or Body Wave

The correct length for hair that is to be permed is long enough for the hair to wrap around the perm rod to be used (different color rods vary in size) at least two-and-a-half times minimum. This length will ensure the rod's position during the perming process and gives enough length for curl retention. There is no maximum length.

Cut hair as evenly as possible to allow for ease of rolling.

If there is enough length, leave the hair at least one-third longer than the final cut you have in mind. The extra length will allow for the seemingly shrinking or pulling back of the hair after perming and for extra shaping the hair probably will need after the perm. Also for cutting off frizzed ends from improper rolling.

This is one time thinning shears are not used. Using thinning shears will cause some short hairs to stick out of the rods while the perm is processing, causing an improper result.

7

Feature Cuts

In the pages that follow we feature some sample cuts in different lengths and styles. We sometimes combine techniques that you have learned previously.

As you get more efficient in your haircutting and as you learn to really look into the flow of hair and what looks best on a client, you will be able to mix and match techniques on your own. But for now, stick to the instructions and illustrations coming up.

As on all haircuts, use your imagination to create. So as not to confuse you with the sectioning, for layered haircuts we will use letters for the different sections, and for one-length cuts we will use numbers.

Little Boy's Cut

Layered, cut short on sides and back with feathered bangs, this style is a carefree cut for a child. It is a basic layered cut.

Section A

Start with back right of section A. Lift hair out and away from head to cut (ninety-degree rule). Section and cut across all of section A.

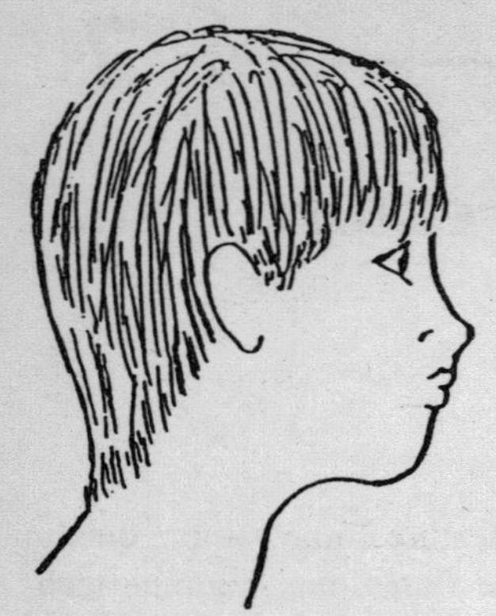

Little boy's cut

Section B

Cut from right to left. Pick up a bit of section A for length comparison with each section strip.

Section C

Cut right to left. Blend with section B and angle short at bottom.

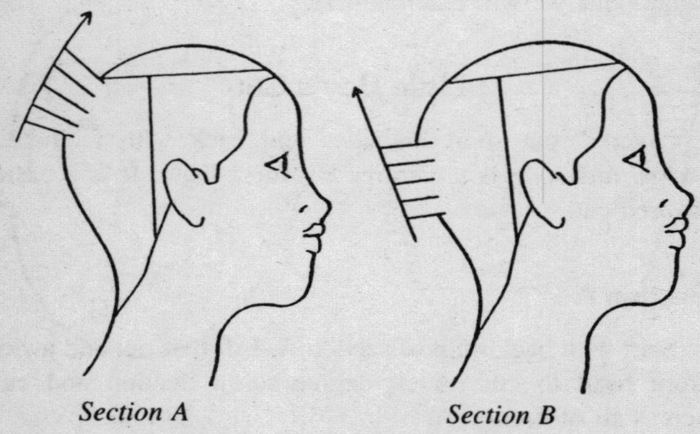

Section A *Section B*

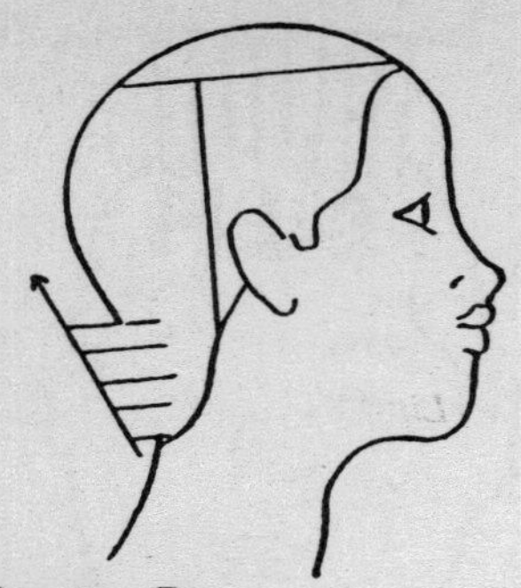

Section C

Section D

Comb away section E. Cut section D from front to back, to and into sections B and C, angling short at bottom.

Section E

Comb away side cap. Comb section E down over section D. Cut section E to and into sections A and B. Comb hair forward at front of sections D and E, and trim off excess.

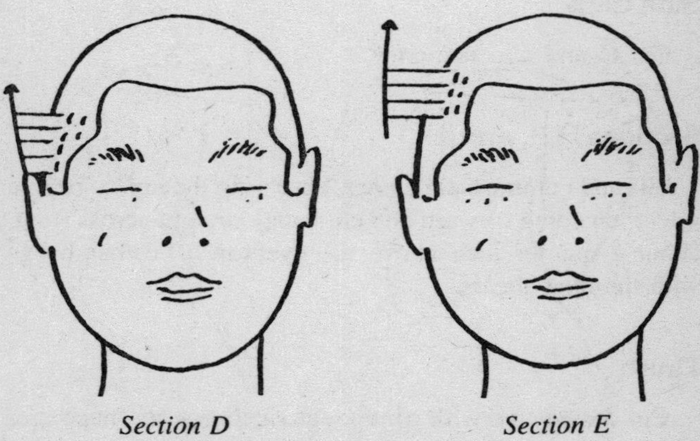

Section D *Section E*

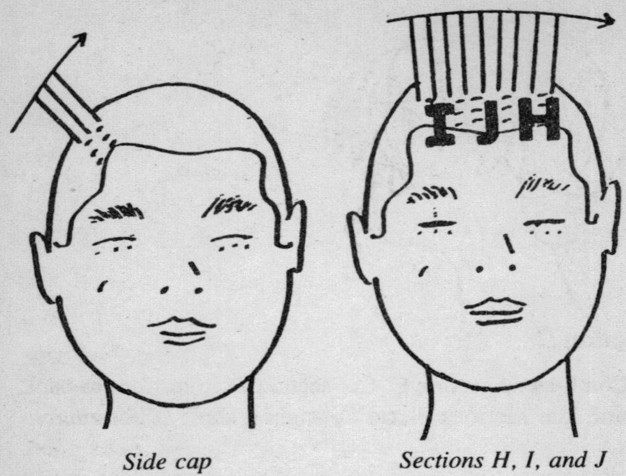

Side cap   *Sections H, I, and J*

Sections F and G

Same procedure as sections D and E.

Side Caps

Cut to and into section A.

Sections H, I, and J

Lift and cut in usual manner, observing the ninety-degree rule, then comb forward and cut bangs straight across front, about a quarter inch above the eyebrows. Feather bangs with thinning shears.

Finish

Cut design line with trimmer at sideburns and nape area of neck. Trim off excess at nape.

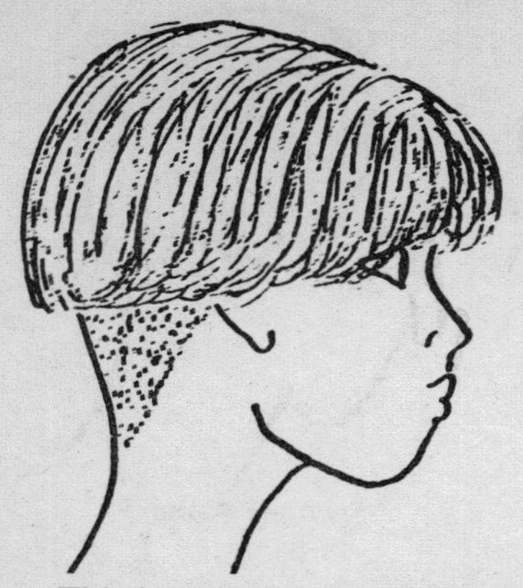

Children's style

Children's Style

This is a short, one-length cut with ridged back and convertible bangs. If this cut gets messed, it still looks good. There must be enough length for all hair to reach the design line to be classified as a one-length cut. However, it can be cut on layered hair and allowed to grow into a one-length design.

Sections 1, 2, and 3

Comb or clip away all sections except sections 1, 2, and 3.

With your #2 blade placed against the skin at the right lower nape area, raise the blade flat to the scalp, even in line with the top of the ear, all across section 1.

Sections 4 and 5

Comb section 4 down over buzzed area and cut a design line with your scissors all across back section, even in line to about a quarter of the way lower than the top of the ear. This design line must hang over buzzed area at least a half inch.

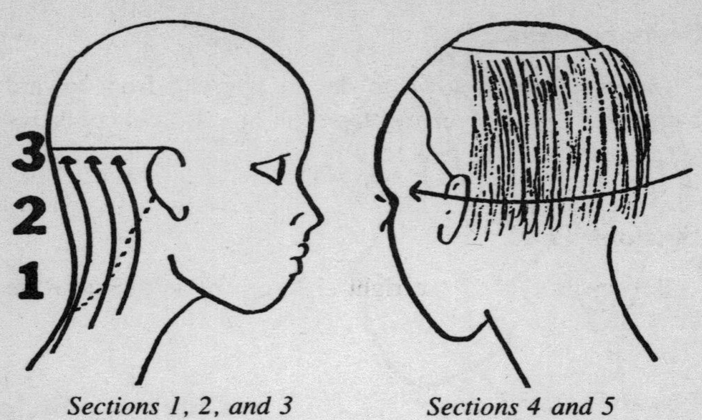

Sections 1, 2, and 3 *Sections 4 and 5*

Section 6

Comb away above sections. Comb section 6 straight down and cut a design line about a quarter inch lower than the top of the ear to meet with the back section design line.

Sections 7 and 8

Comb section 7 down and cut even with design line, followed by section 8.

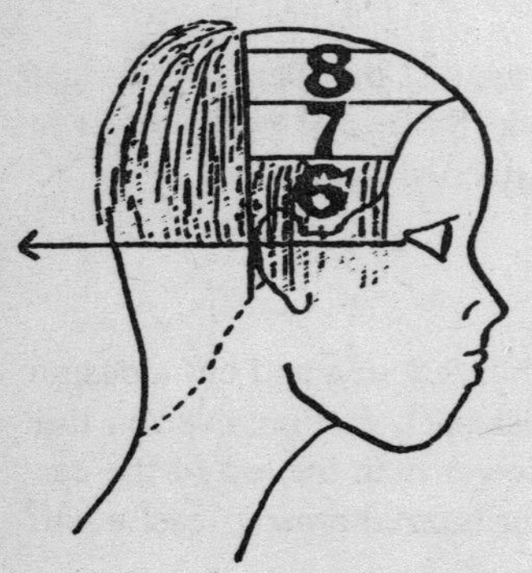

Sections 6, 7, and 8

Sections 9 and 10

Comb section 9 down to design line and front toward bang area. Cut side even with design line. Do not cut bangs yet. Repeat with section 10.

Sections 11 to 15

Repeat process of the right side, on the left side of the head.

Lower Design Line

Use trimmer to cut a sharp design line along the bottom and sides of nape area.

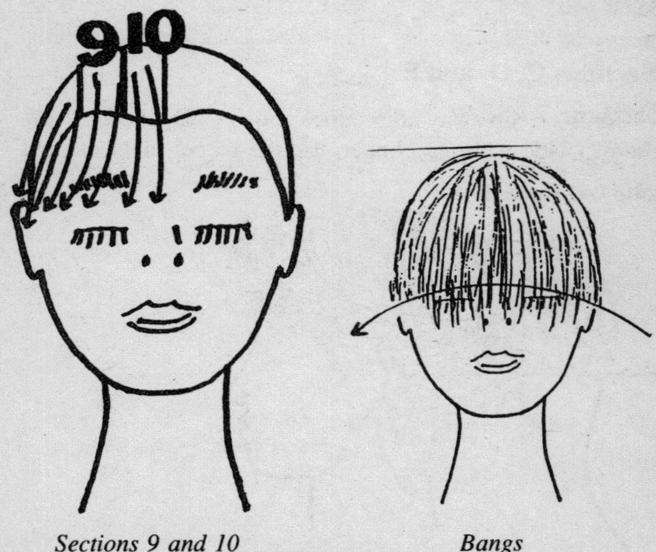

Sections 9 and 10

Bangs

Bangs

Comb top section forward, cut bangs at eyebrow to a quarter inch above.

Blow-Dry

This cut can be finished blown all forward at front. Optionally, after drying forward, brush and blow bangs back and let fall, coax left or right.

Long Layered Top, Tapered Back and Sides

The *GQ* look is good for straight or wavy hair. Shampoo, towel-dry hair, and brush it back. Let it fall. That's all it takes to keep this cut and still look cool. The long layers of this cut must be about five inches to seven inches long.

Sections C, D, and F

Comb or clip away all sections above C, D, and F. Using the #2 blade with the clipper, use the barber taper method

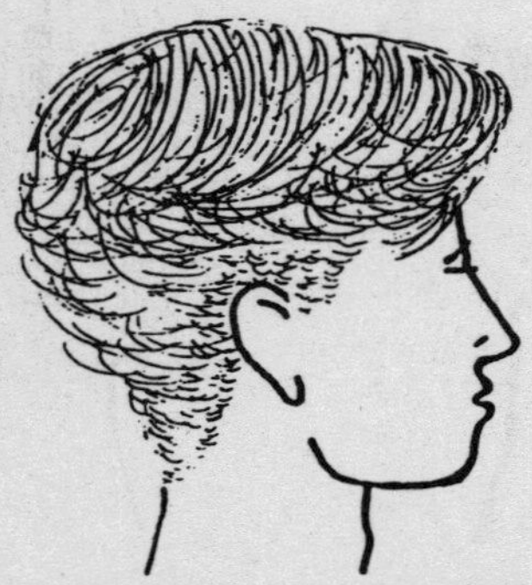

Long layered top, tapered back and sides

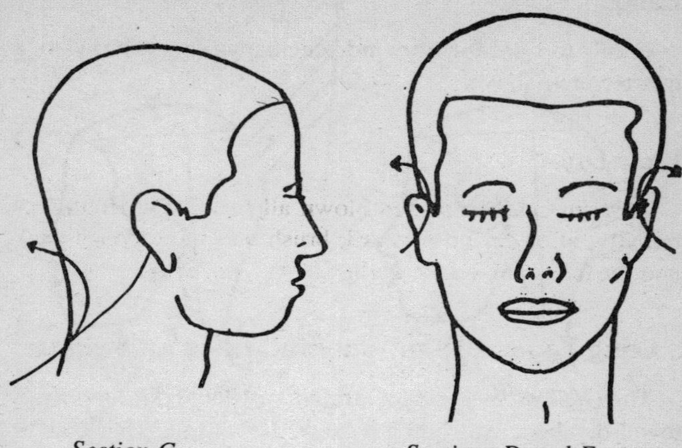

Section C *Sections D and F*

on sections C, D, and F. Keep the taper low, about midway up on the sections.

Section B

Comb or clip away all sections above and forward of section B. Using the section strip method, cut section B from right to left, at the extreme angle shown, blending bottom with section C and leave length at top of section.

Section A

Cut right to left in section strips. Cut section A, picking up a bit of section B for length comparison. Angle section A longer on top.

Section E

Comb or clip away all sections above section E. Cut section E from front to back with the section strip method

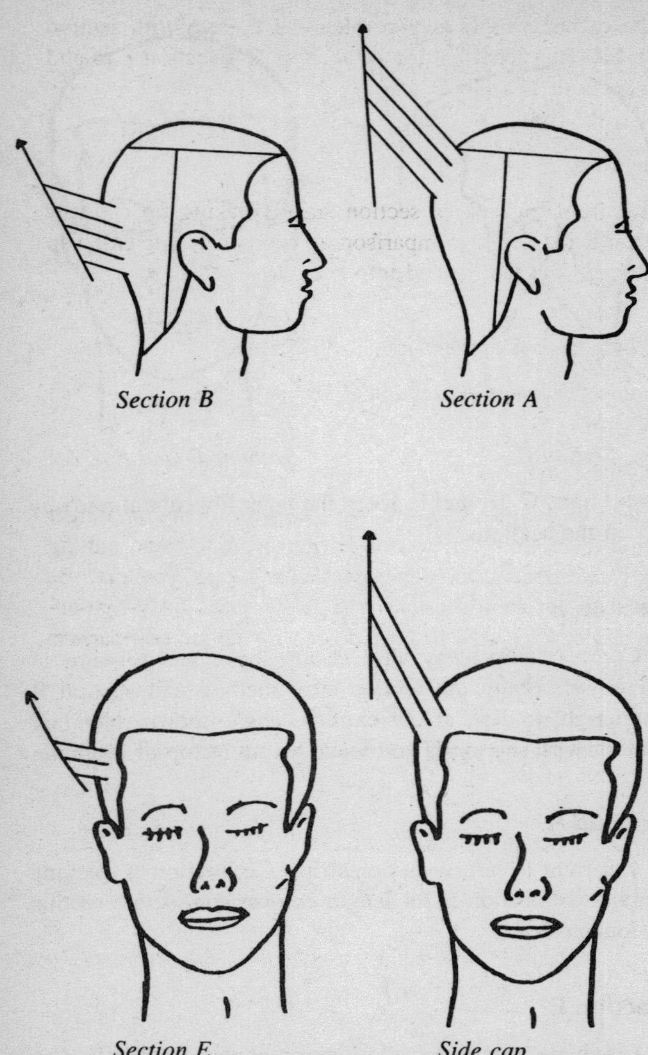

Section B

Section A

Section E

Side cap

at the extreme angle shown, blending bottom with section D and leaving length at top of section. Cut section E to and into sections B and C.

Side Cap

Cut front to back in section strips, picking up a bit of section E for length comparison as you cut. Angle side cap longer on top. Cut to and into section A.

Section G and Side Cap

Same procedure as section E and side cap.

Section H

The top sections are left five to seven inches or longer at your discretion. Cut section H from front to back, pulling hair forward at a forty-five-degree angle as you cut. Be careful to cut each section strip at the same forty-five-degree angle. Pick up a bit of side cap for length comparison as you cut.

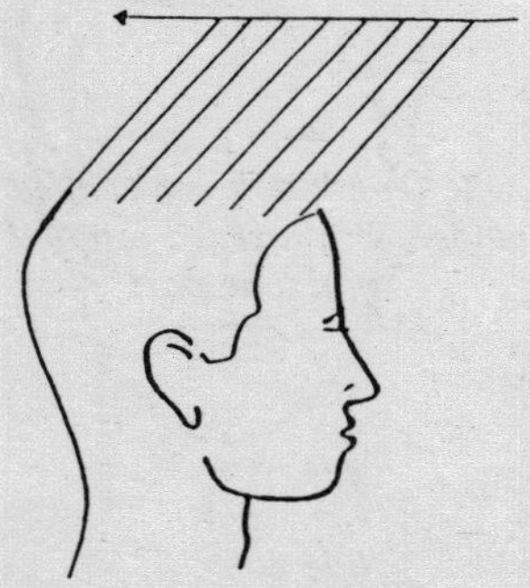

Section H

Sections I and J

Cut at the same angle as section H.

Blend

Blend using thinning shears, with scissors over comb method. Blend hair at sides and back where short meets long. Extreme blending is not essential with this cut.

Design Line

Cut design line with trimmer at sides and nape area.

Maintain

Wear natural, or with gel or pomade for a wet look.

One-Length Bob Cut Cupped Under with Layered Top and Right Side Part (Girl)

This cut can be done in many different ways. It looks great when left all one length with no layers or when

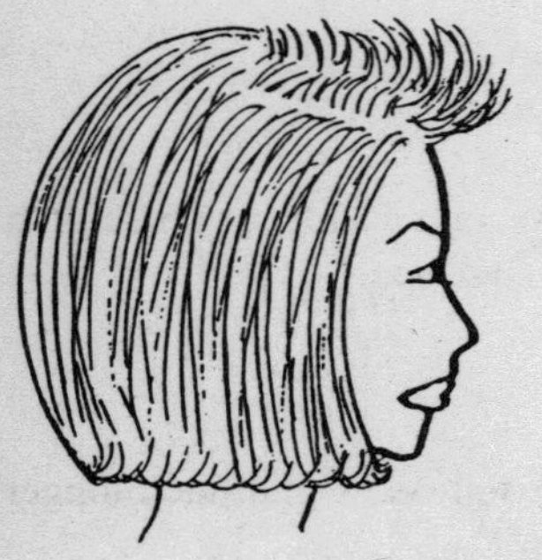

One-length bob cut cupped under with layered top and right side part

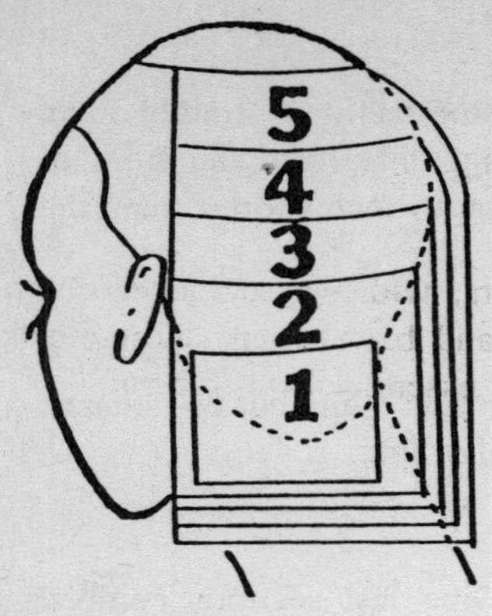

Sections 1 to 5

permed with tight or loose curls. When done with curls, it is best in a blunt cut.

Section 1

Section and clip away all sections except section 1. Comb section 1 straight down and cut a design line halfway up the neckline, a half inch shorter than the final length desired.

Section 2

Comb section 2 down over section 1 and cut one eighth inch longer than section 1's design line.

Sections 3, 4, and 5

Sections 3, 4, and 5 are each left one eighth inch longer than the previous section.

Section 6

Clip away sections 7 to 10. Comb section 6 straight down at the angle shown. Cut a design line from the front of section 6 to, but three-quarters of an inch shorter than, the back section design line.

Section 7

Comb section 7 down over section 6 and cut one quarter inch longer than section 6's design line.

Sections 8 and 9

Sections 8 and 9 should be the last sections combed down and cut in on the right side. Leave sections 8 and 9 long enough to be even with the back section design line. Make sure you leave each section longer than the previous one to allow for the cupping technique.

Section 10

Do not cut section 10 at this time. Section 10 will be cut later when cutting the top.

Section 11

Clip away sections 12 to 15. Comb section 11 straight down. Cut a design line to match section 6's design line angle, but three-quarters of an inch shorter than the back section design line.

Section 12

Comb section 12 down over section 11 and cut one quarter inch longer than section 11's design line.

Sections 13 and 14

Sections 13 and 14 should be the last sections combed down and cut in on the left side. Leave sections 13 and 14

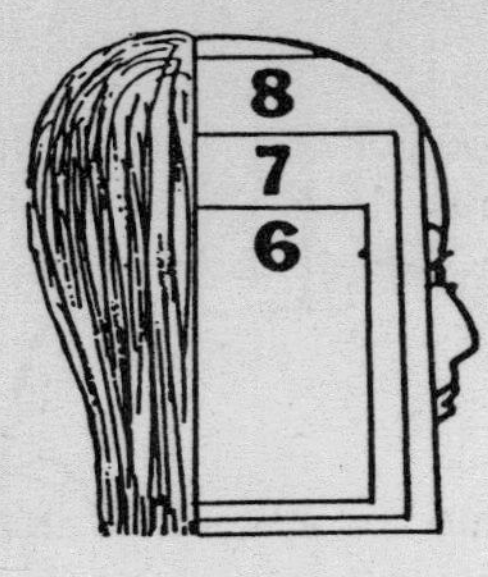

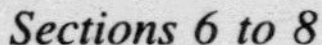

Sections 6 to 8

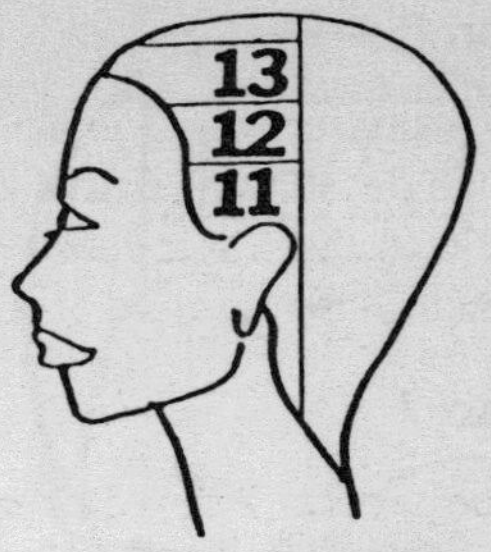

Section 11

long enough to be even with the back section design line. Make sure you leave each section longer than the previous one to allow for the cupping technique.

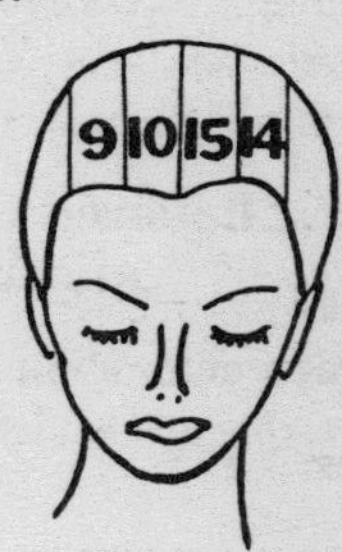

Sections 9, 10, 14, and 15

Top

At this time, put a second part parallel to the first. Comb top straight back and cut in section strips from four inches to six inches long, depending on the length you prefer, back and into the crown area. Thin top only, as needed. These are sections 10 and 15.

Styling

Blow-dry the sides and back with a curling-under motion and a round brush or use a curling iron for stubborn hair. Blow-dry top from right to left and back. When dry, allow front to fall forward.

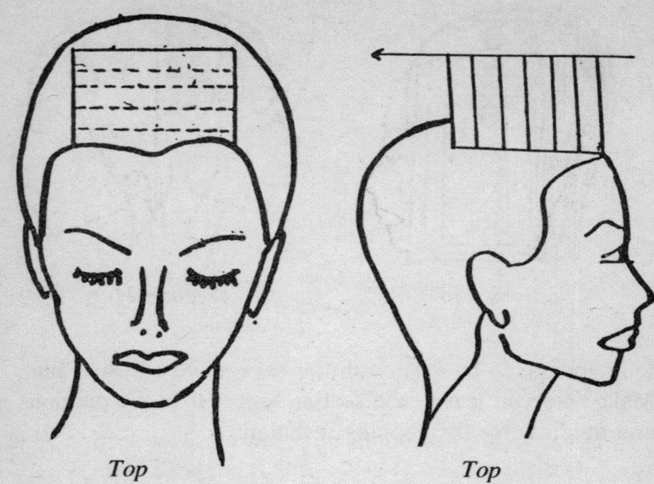

Layered Cut with Feathered Back and Weight on Top (Girl)

This cut is short and easy to keep. It can be quickly blown-dry and styled for people on the go.

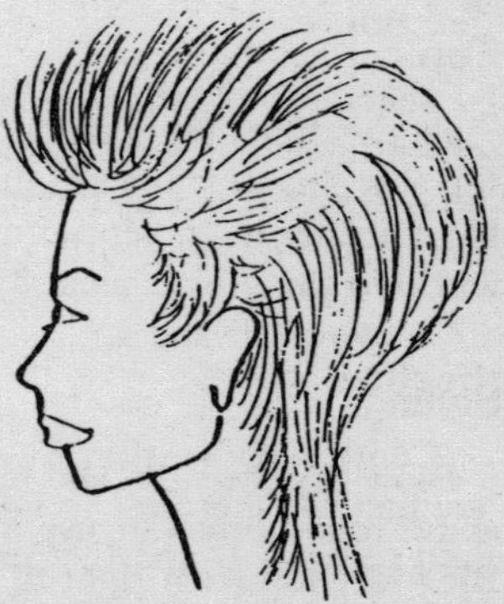

Layered cut with feathered back and weight on top

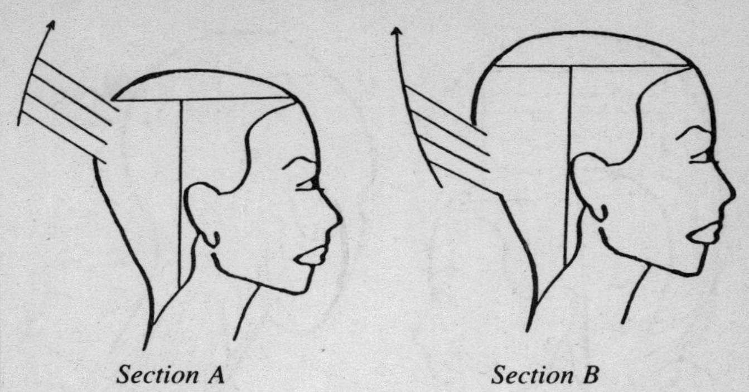

Section A *Section B*

Section A

Start with the back right of section A. Cut section A in section strips all across section A at angle shown.

Section B

Cut from right to left. Pick up a bit of section A for length comparison with each section strip.

Section C

Section C is cut in two steps. The first is about halfway down into the nape area, leaving the lower half long. The second part is cut approximately three inches to five inches long and a design line is cut in. This area is then feathered.

Section D

Comb away section E and the hair above. Cut section D angling for shortness at bottom, from front to back, to and into sections B and C. Comb section D straight down and

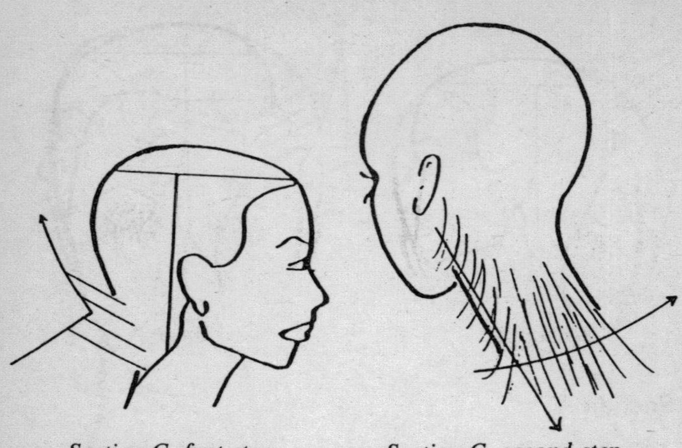

Section C, first step *Section C, second step*

cut a design line around the ear. Use the scissors over comb method to shorten hair around the ear, if necessary.

Section E

Cut to and into sections A and B at angle shown.

Side Cap

Cut to and into back at angle shown.

Sections F and G

Same procedure as sections D and E and side cap.

Section H

Cut section H from front to back, pulling hair forward at a forty-five-degree angle as you cut. Be careful to cut each section strip at the same forty-five-degree angle.

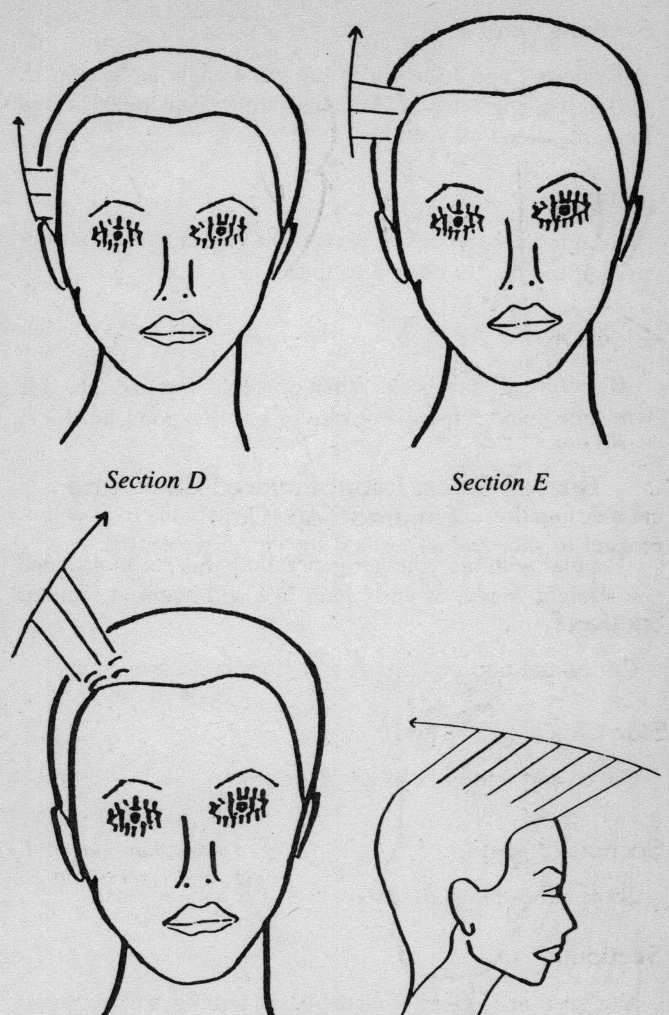

Section D

Section E

Side cap

Section H

Sections I and J

Sections I and J are cut at the same angle as section H. Check top angle by holding hair from front to back and forward. Blend all sections.

Thinning

Thin top section in two parts if the hair is thin or in three parts if the hair is normal to thick.

Blow-Dry

Blow-dry all hair back. When dry, coax top to either side with brush and fingers. Pomade or gel is a good finish.

Buzzed Sides, Long, Layered Back, and Layered Top (Guy)

Popular with the younger generation, this cut looks good on straight, wavy, or curly hair. We will begin at sections D and F.

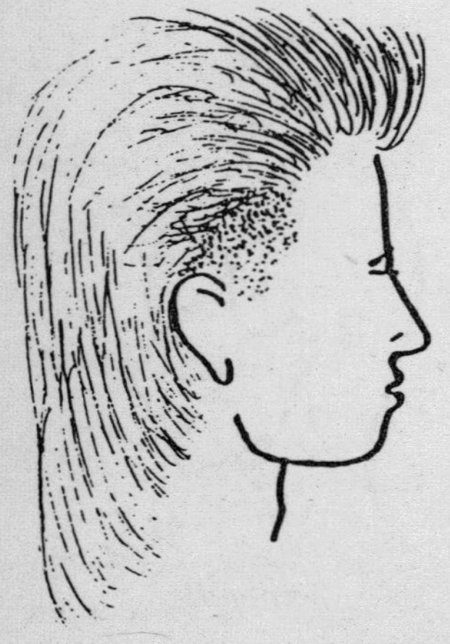

Buzzed sides, long, layered back, and layered top

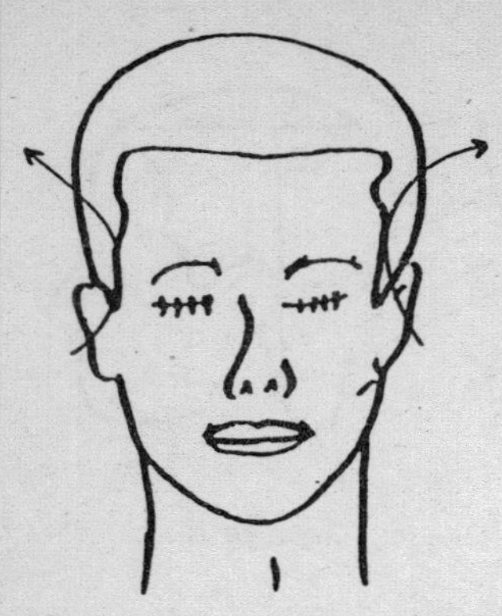

Sections D and F

Sections D and F

Using the barber taper method, with a #2 blade, taper about halfway up the sides at the front of sections D and F, gradually tapering toward the back lower and lower, until you reach midway to the end of the ear.

Optional: Taper this section with the #1 blade after the #2 blade for additional closeness.

Section A

Start with the back right of section A. Cut section A in section strips all across section A at diagonal shown.

Section B

Cut from right to left. The same diagonal applies. Use section A as a guide and cut to match angle.

Section C

Cut section C at the same angle as sections A and B. Tilt the head forward and cut a design line across the bottom

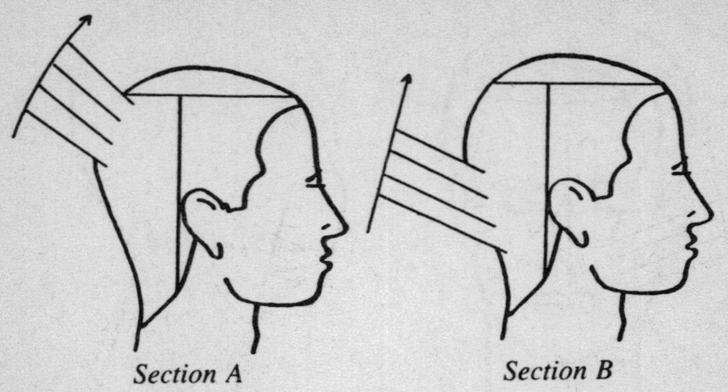

Section A

Section B

of section C. Lift the head, curve sides of section C toward the front, and cut a design line at sides. Blend side and bottom design lines.

Section E

Comb section E down over already buzzed section D. Cut section E in section strips to and into sections A and B, blending section E with section D as you cut.

Sections F and G

Cut sections F and G in the same manner as sections D and E.

Side Caps

Cut to and into back section at angle shown.

Sections H, I, and J

Cut sections H, I, and J in section strips from front to back, blending with side caps and section A.

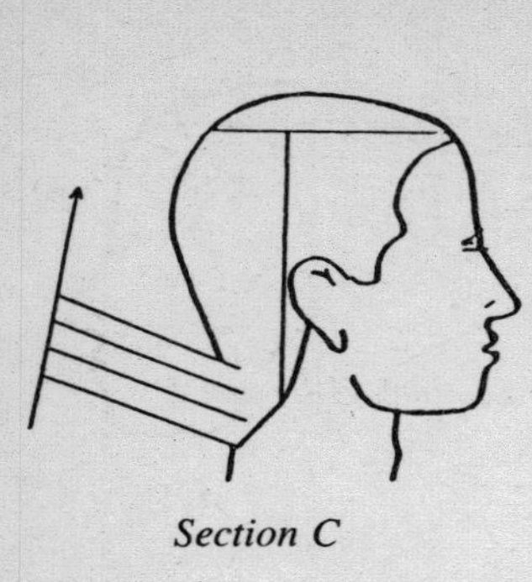

Section C

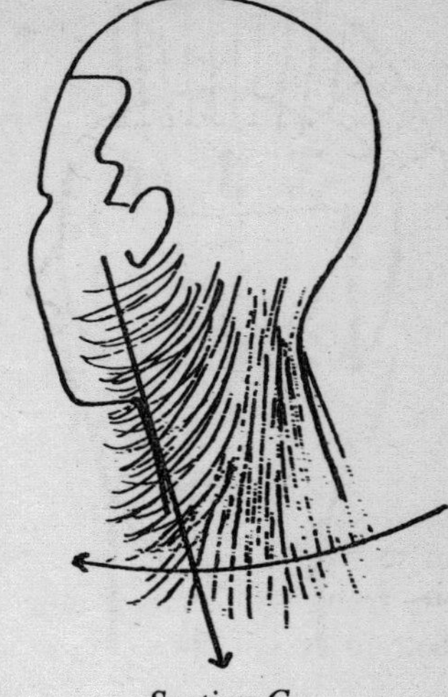

Section C

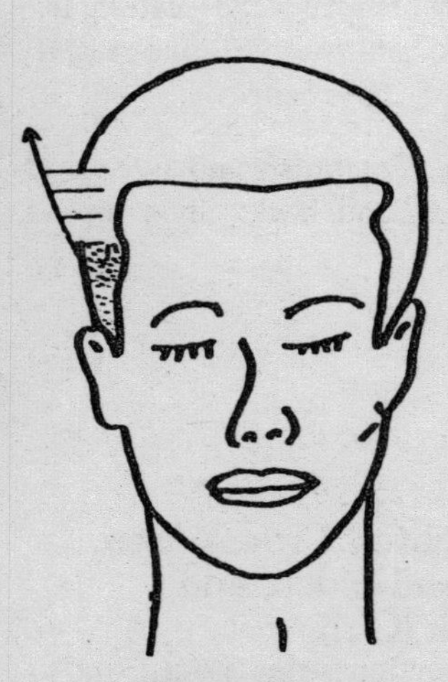

Section E

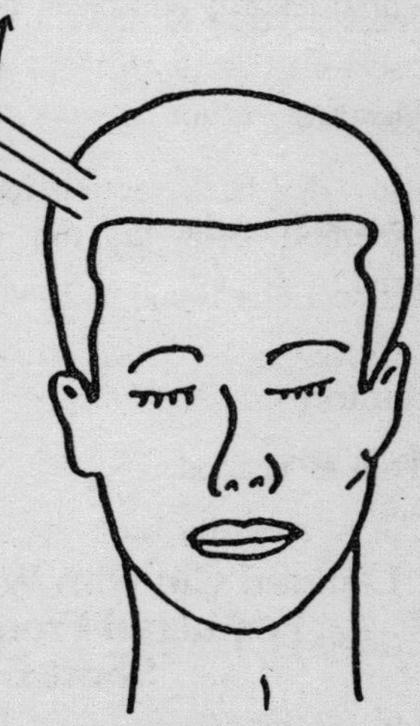

Side cap

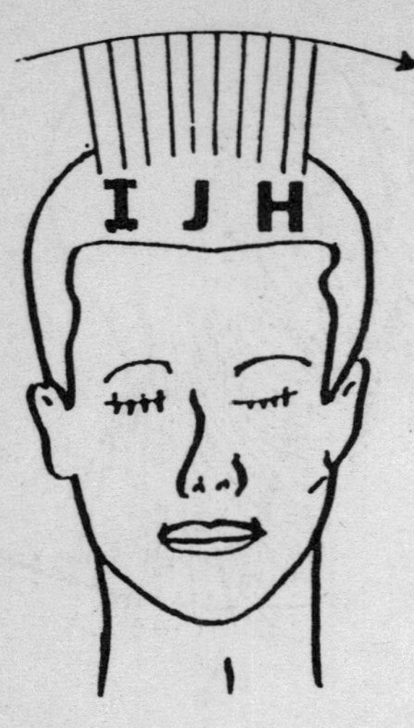

Sections H, I, and J

Finish

Cut sideburns and clean neck with trimmer.

Blow-Dry

Blow-dry back section using vent brush and twist and lift method. Blow-dry top, sides, and back. Style top as desired.

Thinning

Thin as needed.

Layered Cut with Weight at Crown Area, Feathered Front and Sides, and Short Back (Girl)

A wash and wear casual cut, it's easy to maintain.

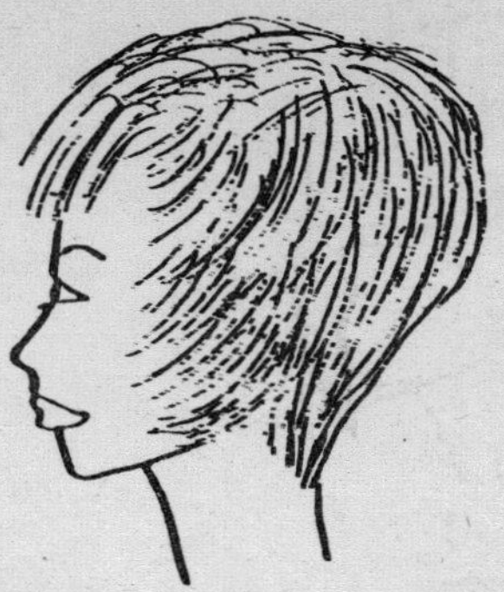

Layered cut with weight at crown area, feathered front and sides, and short back

Section A

Start with the back right of section A. Cut section A in section strips all across section A at angle shown.

Section B

Cut from right to left. Cut section B into converging angle of section A.

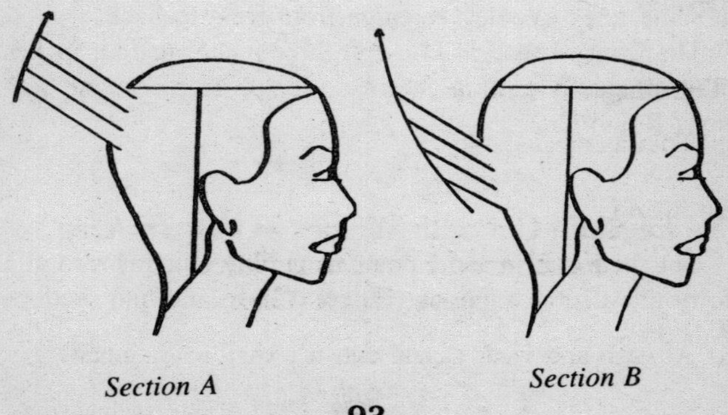

Section A *Section B*

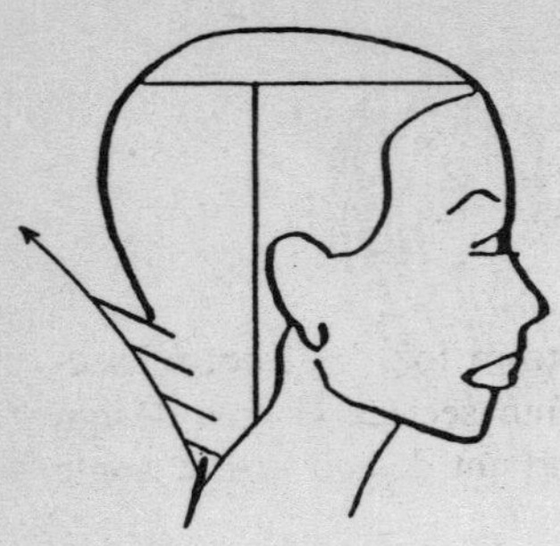

Section C

Section C

Section C is cut as close as you can get it with your fingers to the nape.

Design Line

Cut design line at nape area. Finish design line with trimmer.

Section D

Section D is cut in section strips, pulling hair forward at a forty-five degree angle as you cut. Cut each section strip at same forty-five-degree angle from front to back.

The front of section D is left three inches to four inches long, gradually getting shorter in length to meet with sections B and C.

Section E

Cut section E in same manner, pulling hair forward at a forty-five-degree angle as you cut. Cut to and into sections A and B.

Section F and G

Cut in the same manner as sections D and E.

Design Line

Side design line is cut going from long at front of sections D and F, to short at and into section B area design line. Curve sides toward front and cut design line at angle shown.

Side Caps

Cut side caps in section strips. Cut front of side cap one-and-a-half inches shorter than top section of section A. Side cap gradually gets longer at each section strip until it meets with section A.

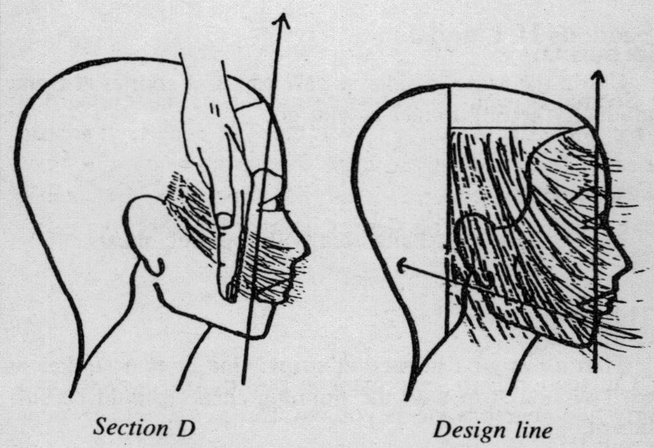

Section D *Design line*

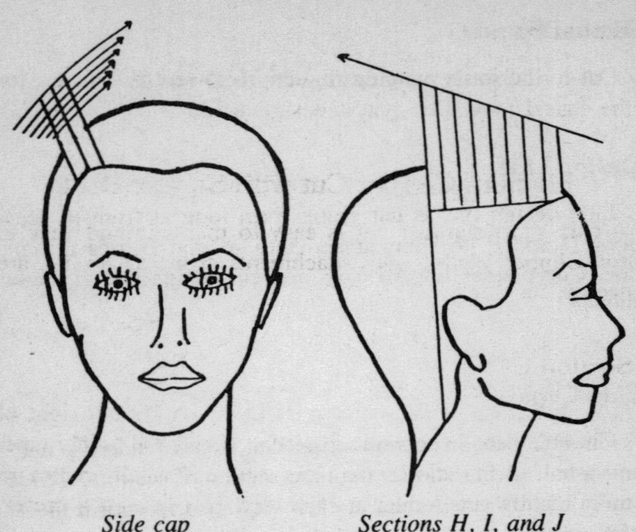

Side cap

Sections H, I, and J

Sections H, I, and J

Cut in the same manner as side cap. Cut shorter at front, gradually getting longer as you go.

Feathering

Feather sides and bang area with thinning shears.

Thinning

Thin all around in section strips. One or two strokes at each section strip with the thinning shears should be sufficient.

Blow-Dry

Use vigorously moving fingers, followed by blower, for the casual look this style is designed for.

Medium Clipper Cut with Square Back

This short summer cut is easy to maintain and easy to do. Clipper blades and attachments from #1 to #4 are needed for this cut.

Section C

With the #2 blade, start your cut at the bottom right of section C, below the natural hairline. Using the barber taper method, raise the clipper from one-and-a-half inches to three inches (depending on how high of a taper you prefer) all across section C.

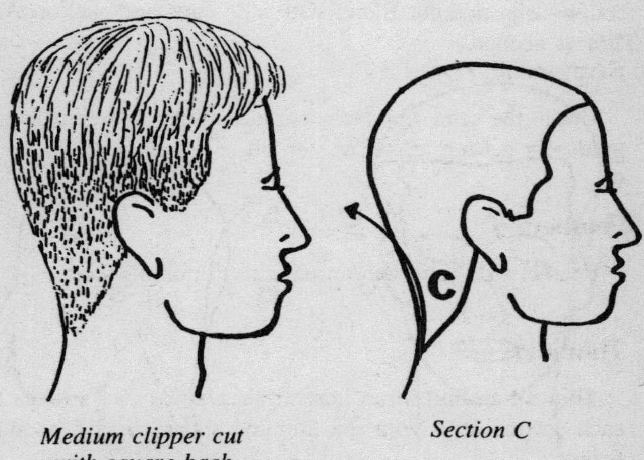

Medium clipper cut with square back

Section C

Sections D and F

Repeat previous process on sections D and F.

Sections B and A

With the head up and level all around, place the #4 clipper attachment against the scalp. Cut section B straight up into section A and out of the cut with a continuous motion. (Do not run clipper against the scalp at the top of the stroke; gradually ease it out.)

Sections E, G, and Side Caps

Repeat previous process on sections E, G, and side caps.

Sections H, I, and J

Cut these sections one inch to three inches in section-section-strip method. Blend with side caps and section A. Thin as needed.

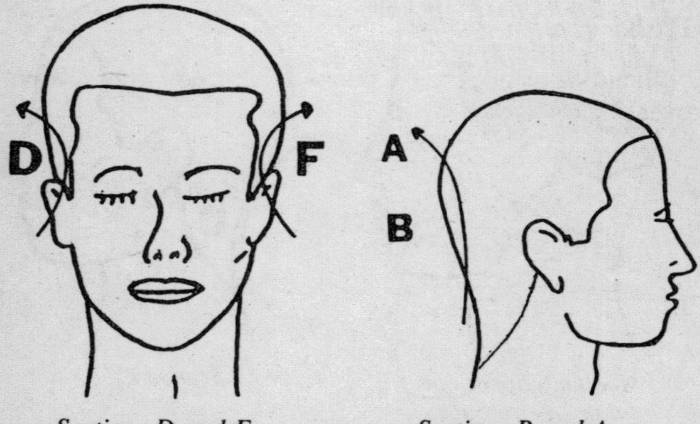

Sections D and F　　*Sections B and A*

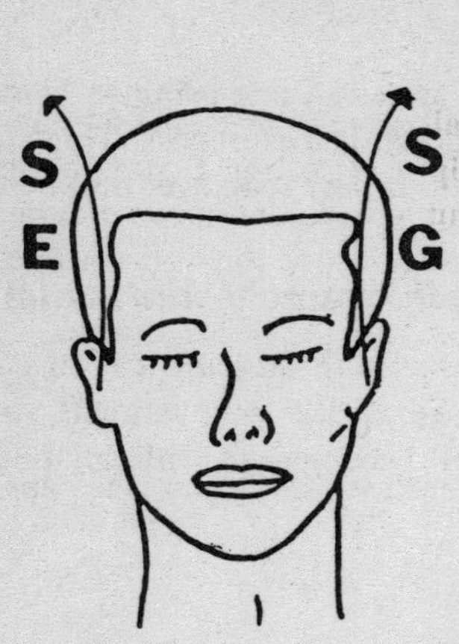

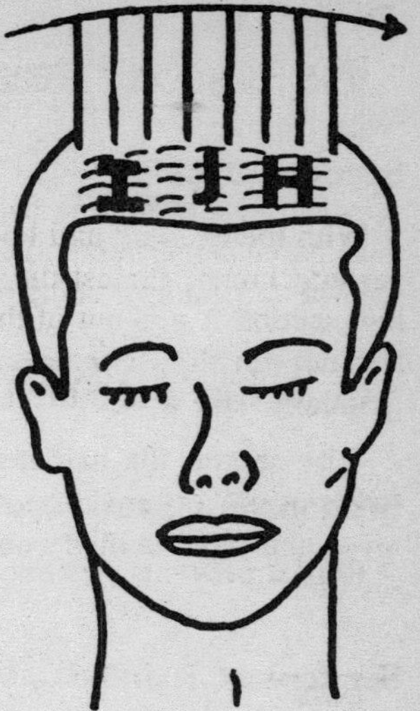

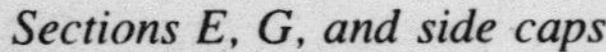

Sections E, G, and side caps

sections H, I, and J

Blend

Blend all converging sections, if needed, with scissors over comb method.

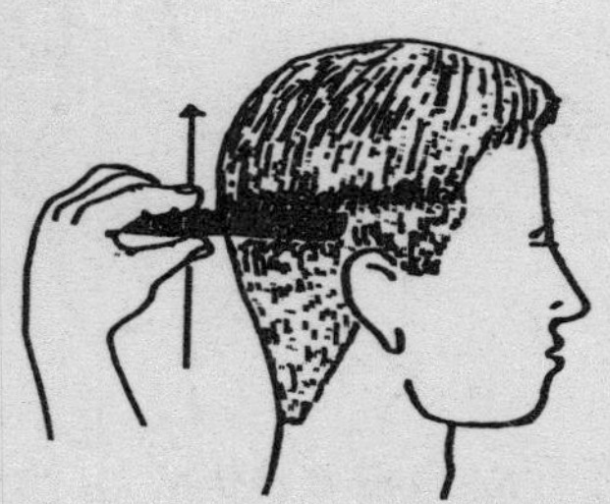

Blend

Design Line

Cut a design line at sideburns around ears and nape area with trimmer.

Optional: Cut bottom fringe at design line using #1 blade and barber taper method for additional closeness. This cut can be left long or short on top or any length in between.

Crew Cut and Flat Top (Extremely short cuts)

The shorter the hair gets, the more difficult it is to cut without making mistakes. However, the more haircuts you give, the more skilled you will become—as with anything in life.

Tools

Clipper, #000 blade, #1 blade, #2 blade. Crew cut attachments that fit over the clipper size #3, size #4, flat top rake.

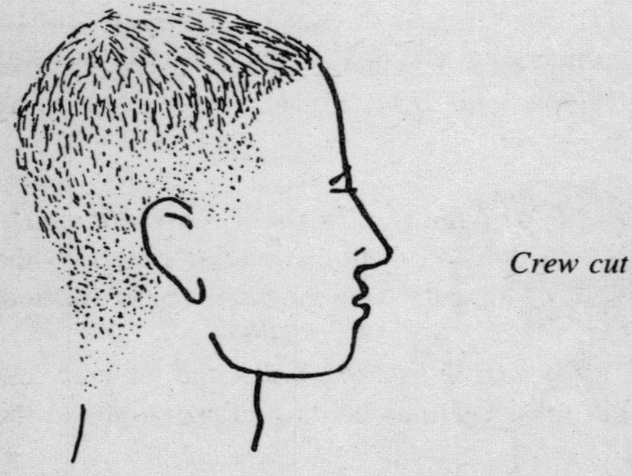

Crew cut

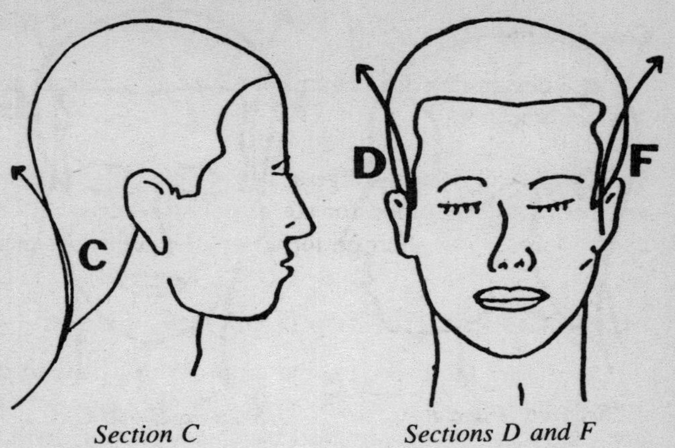

Section C   Sections D and F

The crew cut is by far the easier of the two cuts described here. If the hair is longer (over five inches), give a basic layered haircut down to about three inches all around.

Crew Cut

Sections C, D, and F: Use the #2 blade. Cut these sections starting below the natural hairline, using the barber taper method (see clipper cuts, page 35). Cut these sections up about three inches.

Sections B, A, E, and G: Clip on the #3 crew cut attachment over the #000 blade. Cut these sections up to the higher elevations of the cut, using the barber taper method.

Sections H, I, J, and side cap: Using the #4 crew cut attachment, cut these sections holding clipper right to the scalp.

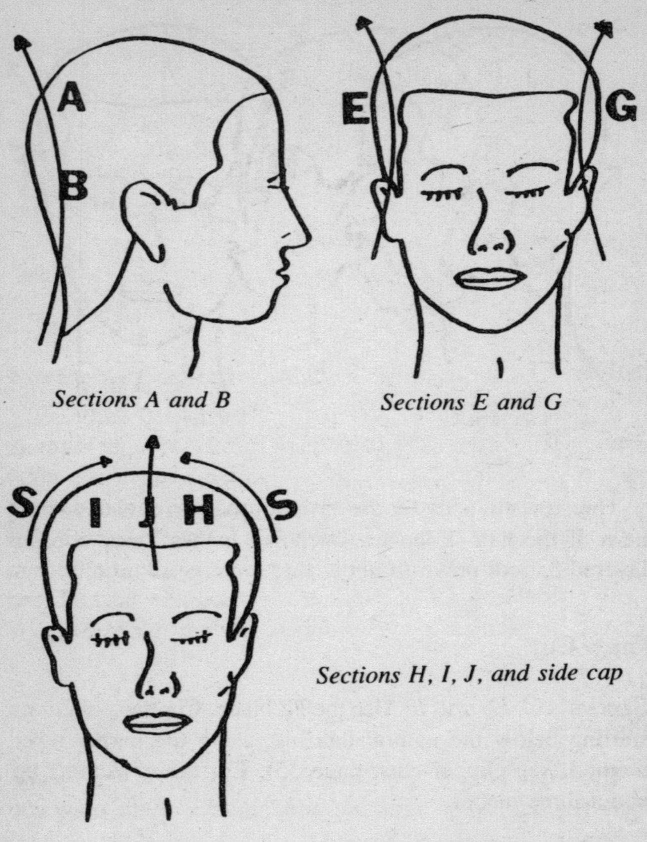

Sections A and B

Sections E and G

Sections H, I, J, and side cap

Blend: Blend all sections using scissors over comb method.

At this point, you can go one of two ways:

Option 1: Cut a design line with your trimmer at the bottom perimeter of the haircut. Clean neck with trimmer. The cut is complete.

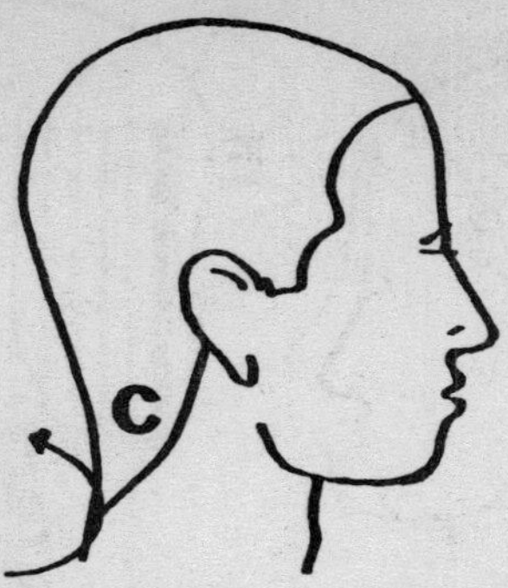

Take the edge off section C with a very light arching upstroke

Option 2: Using the #1 blade with the barber taper method, shorten sections C, D, and F. Attach the #000 blade. Using a very light arching upstroke along the bottom of section C, take the edge off. Cut a design line with your trimmer at the bottom perimeter of the sides of face and neck. Clean neck area with trimmer. The cut is complete.

Flat Top

This style is not recommended for curly or very wavy hair. The flat top is cut in the same manner as the crew cut except for the top.

Follow the directions for the crew cut until you reach Sections H, I, J, and side cap.

Sections H, I, J, and side cap: Comb these sections straight back (dampen if necessary). Make sure head is level all around.

Insert flat top rake from front to back, holding about a

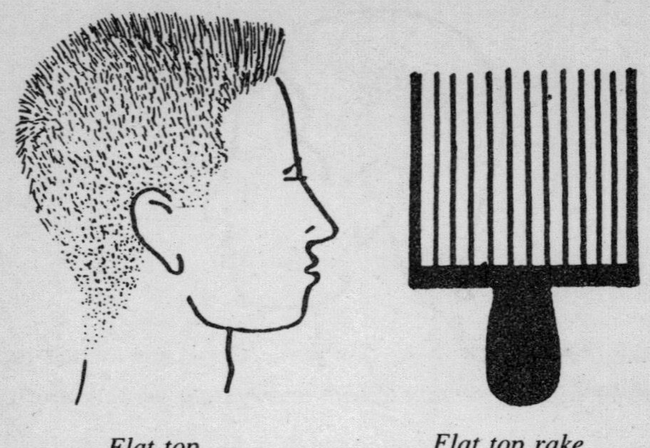

Flat top *Flat top rake*

quarter inch away from top of scalp. Make sure rake is level all around. This will leave the front longer.

Using the #1 blade on clipper, place clipper against rake at back, cut forward to front. Cut all hair sticking out of

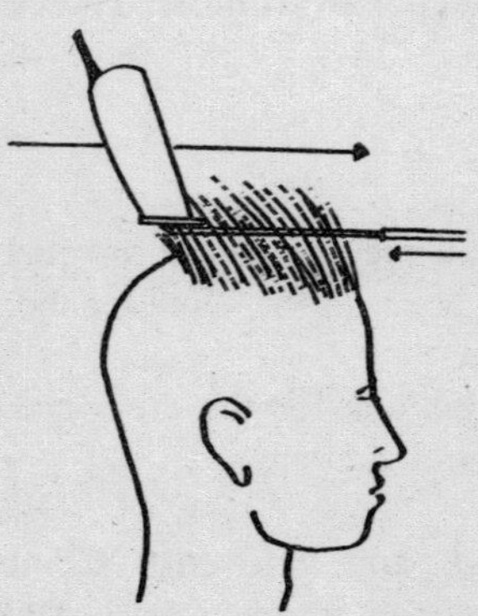

Make sure rake is level all around before clipping hair that sticks out of rake.

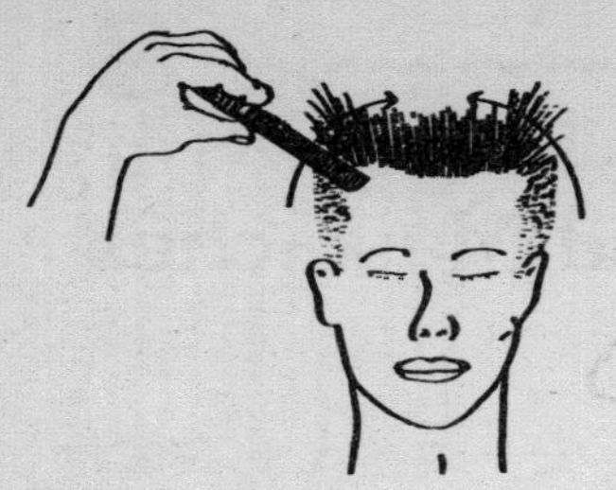

Shape

rake. Remove rake. At this point, the center of the top of the hair should be sticking straight up.

Shape: Shape the top section using the scissors over comb method by combing hair back, and carefully cuting and blending sides, top, and back little by little.

At this point, refer back to instructions for crew cut and start with blend.

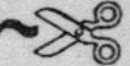 8

Beards and Mustaches

Like haircuts, there are many varieties of beards and mustaches. They can be used to correct the shape of the face, hide a scar, or just add some character.

Beards and mustaches can be used in any combination. When cutting, trimming, and shaping, we can use our clipper with the many different attachments and/or scissors. The ninety-degree rule also applies here.

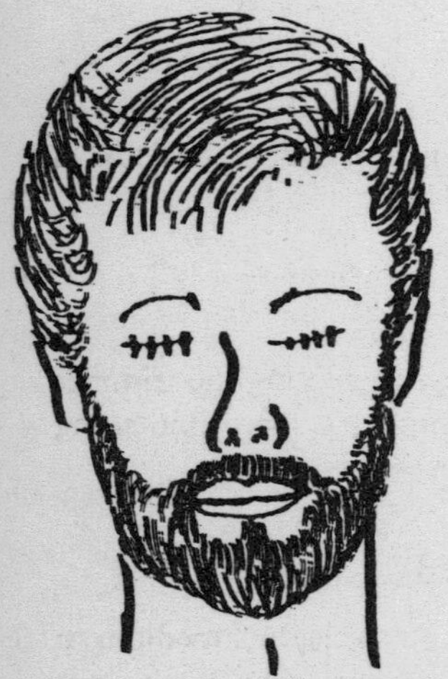

Full Beard and Mustache

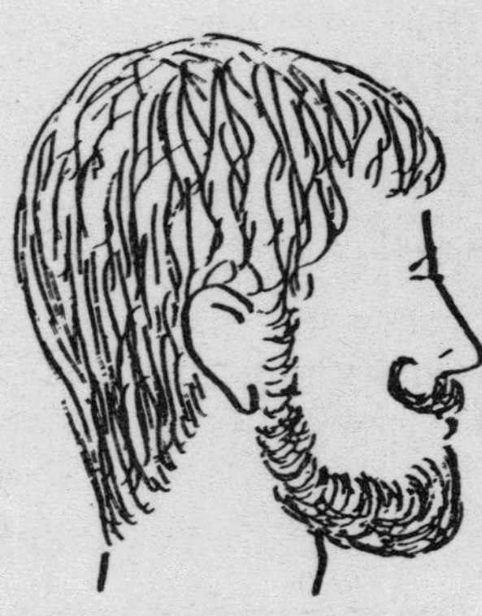

Full Beard with Handlebar Mustache

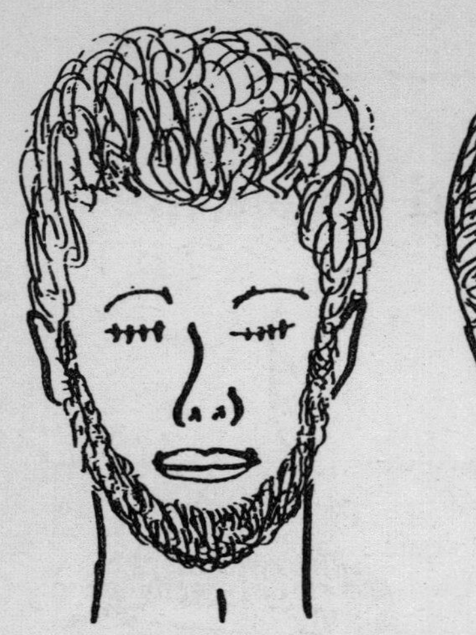

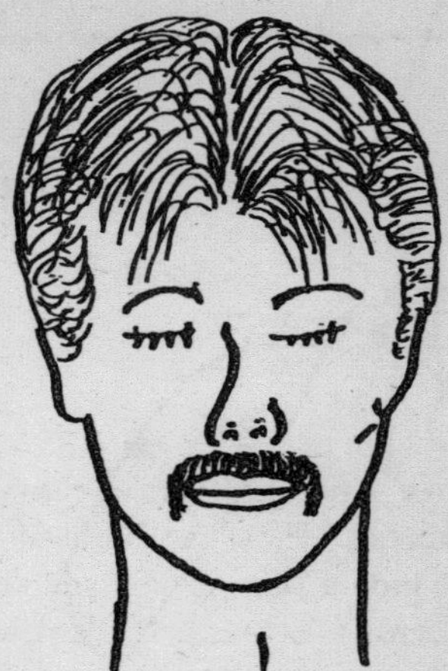

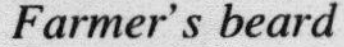

Farmer's beard *Fu Manchu Mustache*

The Mustache

Step 1

Basic mustache trimming is best done with the scissor over comb method. This will reduce the bulk to fullness desired.

Step 2

Follow by combing the hair down, pointing the trimmer blade toward the mustache, and cutting a sharp line along the upper lip line. (See illustration, page 108.)

Full Beard

One of the most popular types of beards, this medium to long length is trimmed using the scissors over comb, sec-

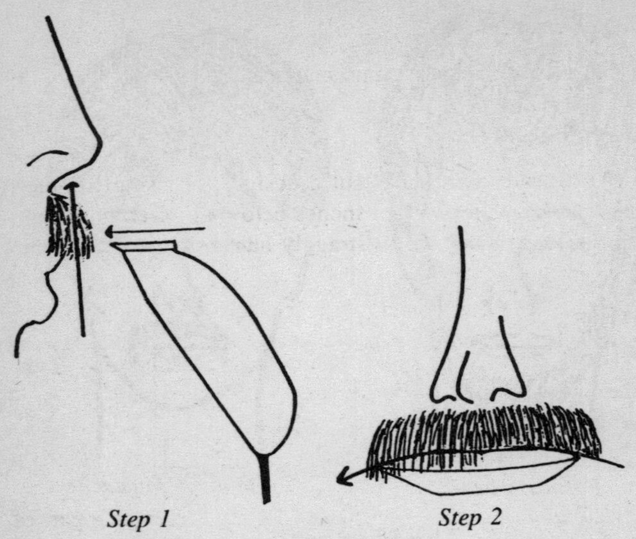

Step 1 *Step 2*

tion strip method. Needing little maintenance, it should be trimmed every three to four weeks. Shape fuller at chin and jaw area, gradually tapering shorter as you get into the neck area to about one-third fullness of longest part of beard.

Section 1

Starting at top center of chin, cut section strips one-and-a-half inches to two inches wide. Cut top to bottom, using scissors over comb method. Cut no more than one quarter inch of length at a time. (Don't forget the ninety-degree rule.)

Sections 2 and 3

Starting at top left of chin, repeat section 1 process, and blend with section 1 as you cut.

Side Sections

Cut side sections in same manner.

Design Line

With head tilted back, cut a design line using trimmer, about three inches to four inches below tip of chin, following contour of jaw. Trim straggly hair around cheek area.

Finish

Use scissors over comb to blend any converging lines. Blend and trim mustache, if any, with beard.

Full Beard, Close Cropped

Use the clipper method, which leaves the longest part of the beard about one inch long.

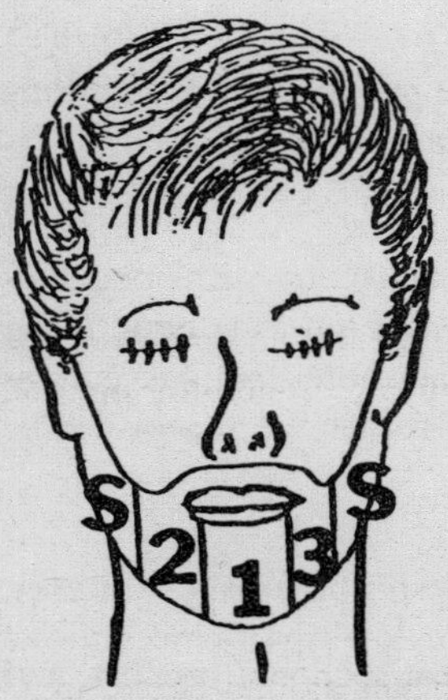

Section strips for beard

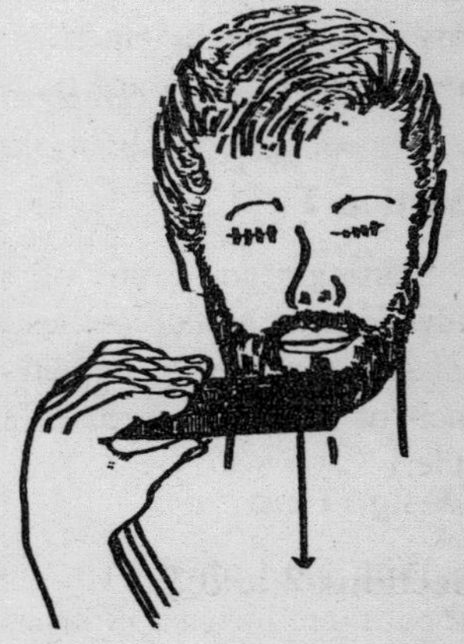

Cut top to bottom, using scissors over comb method

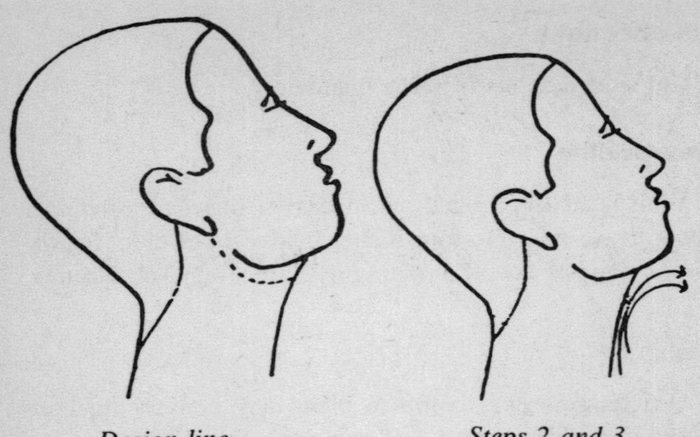

Design line *Steps 2 and 3*

Step 1

Run clipper with attachment #7 along all portions of the beard. Cut from bottom up.

Step 2

Use an arching motion, with clipper attachment #3, along bottom of neck to about one-quarter up the chin.

Step 3

Using the #2 blade, cut along the extreme bottom of the neck, one-quarter of the way up, using an arching motion.

Design Line

With head tilted back, cut a design line using trimmer, about three inches to four inches below tip of chin, following contour of jaw. Trim straggly hair around cheek area.

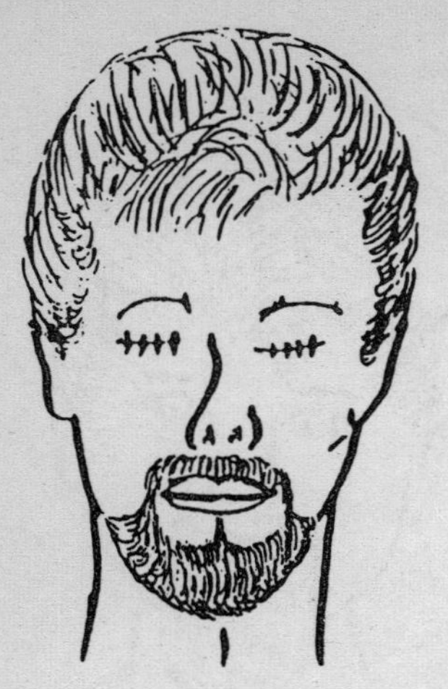

The goatee

The Goatee

Not only used as a facial ornament, this beard is a great way to strengthen a weak chin. It requires a bit more maintenance than a full beard.

Follow the cutting technique for the full beard. With a

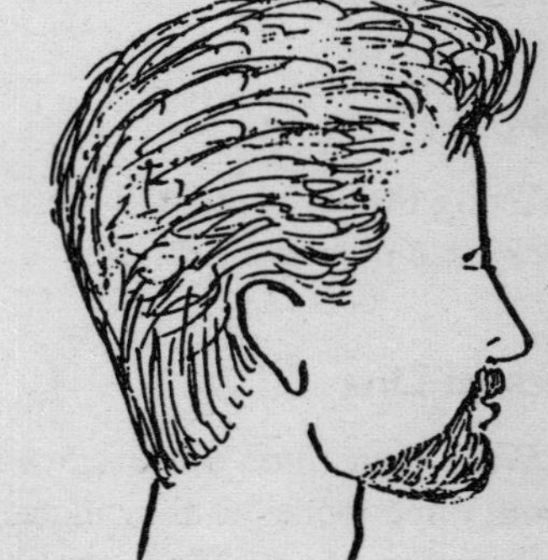

Goatee, side view

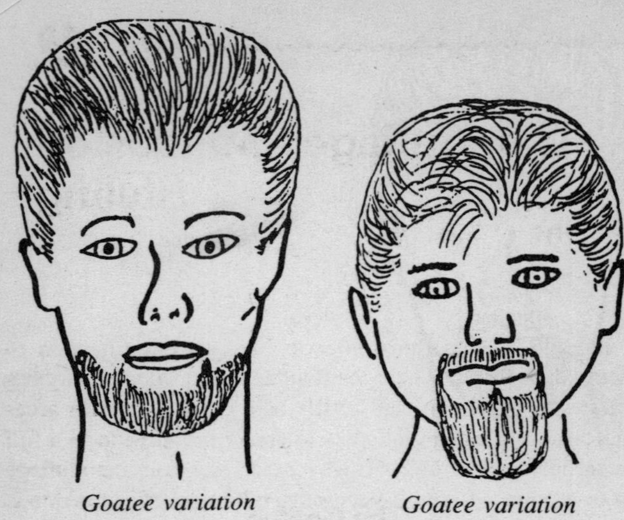

Goatee variation *Goatee variation*

trimmer, slowly cut away unwanted sections. Many variations are possible, depending on the natural hairline and the density of the facial hair.

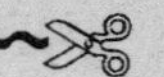 9

Camouflage and Illusion Styling

Balding is something no one likes to have happen to them, and that's where camouflage and illusion styling come into play. We can let the hair grow in certain areas and camouflage the thin spots to create the illusion of a full or partial head of hair. However, we can only camouflage up to a point without it becoming ridiculous. If someone is very bald, with only a strip of hair around the sides and back of his head, it does not work very well or look good when he grows one side very long and combs it over. Instead of the long side staying on top of his head, it's hanging and blowing in the wind most of the time. This sort of person would be better off with a layered cut all around, letting his bald spot show or, if he wants hair that badly, he should get some sort of hair replacement. A good candidate for camouflage and illusion styling is someone with a mild to medium degree of baldness.

Let us determine what sort of illusion style we can create with certain types of heads. The illustrations give you an idea of what different heads look like with all the hair combed straight back. Notice the different degree of baldness on each.

The first illustration shows that the baldness can be somewhat corrected by letting the top front grow and spreading the hair out toward the sides a bit to fill in the temples.

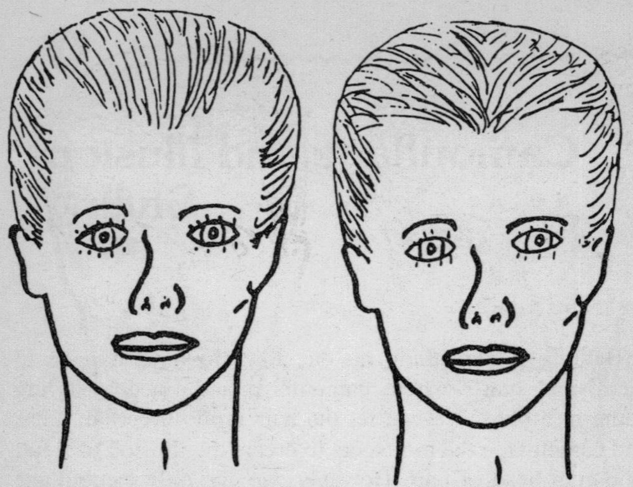

Front hairline missing hair in the temples

Correct by spreading hair out toward the sides

The next illustration shows a head with most of the top hair missing but the sides are not too low for one of them to be grown long and combed over to the opposite side to create an illusion of a full head of hair.

When combing the hair over to the opposite side, for the best results, the long hair has to reach over about one inch to one-and-a-half inches into the other side to hold itself down. Lightly thin in about one inch of the extreme end of the overlap so it meshes with the left side.

The final illustration depicts a crown that area is bald. Here we can go one of two ways. We can use a side part and cover this area as in the previous illustrations, or we can let the front grow long enough and comb the hair back to cover the balding area. Again, let it grow long enough to cover the spot plus one inch to one-and-a-half inches, and lightly thin one inch of the extreme end so it will mesh with the back section.

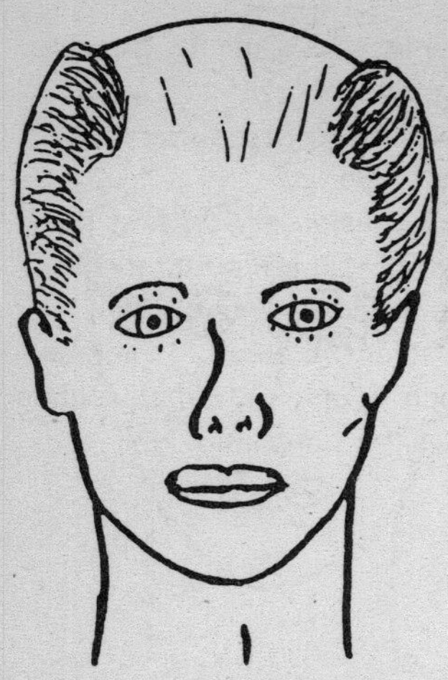

Most of top hair missing

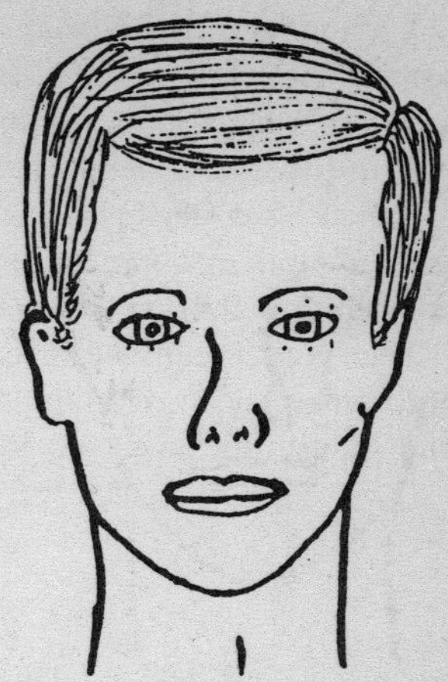

Comb one side across top

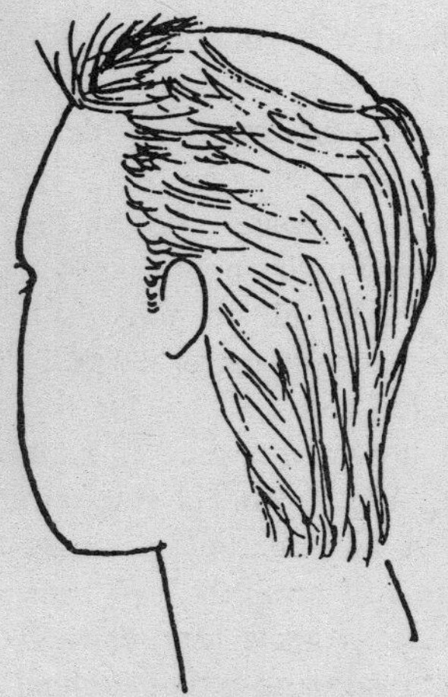

Hair missing from crown

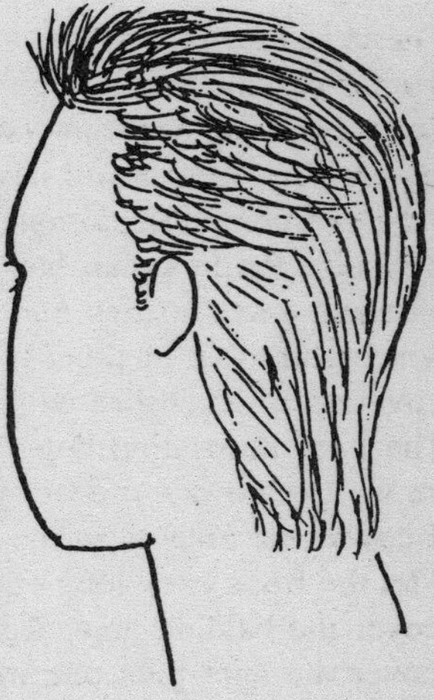

Comb front hair back to cover crown

Camouflage and illusion styling take time to develop, sometimes a few months. Be patient.

If you need styling gel or mousse and hair spray to hold hair in place, use them.

When blow-drying side parted illusion styles, first blow dry the top hair opposite of the way you are going to finish combing the hair. It will lie better and appear fuller.

Use your imagination for different degrees of baldness and remember to overlap one inch to one-and-a-half inches and lightly thin one inch in from the bitter end.

10

Do's and Don'ts

DO:

Think of hair as weight.
Ask questions about overall length, etc.
Take into account the shape of the face when designing a cut.
Start with an idea before you cut. Have the finished product in mind.
Shampoo right before a cut, so the hair will be at its most pliable.
Cut step by step.
Cut using the ninety-degree rule, unless the cut calls for different angles.
Take small sections.
Anticipate shrinking of wet hair.
Use your thinning shears on most haircuts.
Check each section when finished with the basic cut.
Stand behind the client when cutting the top (except when cutting bangs).
Use a mirror as a tool for viewing the overall effect while cutting and styling.
Step away now and then to check the total look.
Use a nylon styling brush.
Give thin hair more layers for added fullness.
Bevel when cutting the back.

DON'T:

- Give a style that goes against the natural flow of the hair.
- Cut blind. Know where the point of the scissors is at all times.
- Cut too wet or too dry. Spray with water if hair starts to dry while cutting.
- Leave hair too long on top when giving a layered cut.
- Chop when cutting scissors over comb. A continuous motion is necessary.
- Cut hair too short around crown or cowlick.
- Cut design line too high above natural hairline (unless the style demands it).
- Overthin.
- Press too hard when trimming with a downstroke.
- Burn hair when blow-drying. Keep it moving.
- Use a natural or close bristle brush while styling.